Yourfitnesssuc

Quick workouts real results

No equipment exercise from beginner to advanced. High-Intensity Bodyweight Workouts for Full-Body Toning and Fat Loss

James Atkinson

Copyright ©

2024 yourfitnesssuccess.com

All rights reserved

Contents

Introduction 1

How to Use This Book 4

Health Check 7

The Importance of Consistency 8

Exercise guidelines 11

Workout length and volume 17

Exercise Cards Explained 19

Workouts 22

Quick Workouts for Busy Schedules 92

Your Workouts Your Way 96

Progression modifiers 101

Some free stuff? 103

Conclusion and Next Steps 104

Blank Exercise Cards 107

Standard 108

Supersets 110

Single exercise 112

The Tonne 114

Video course 116

Introduction

A warm welcome to this fitness and exercise guide!

This fitness book has been written with three major goals in mind. If we, as trainers, or prospective trainers, follow the guide, we will see many positive fitness side effects born from this approach. This is a fast, efficient and effective exercise method!

The three major goals of this book are to:

1. Develop impressive full body fitness, visually and systemically
2. Exclusively use short workout routines (as short as 10 minutes
3. Completely omit workout equipment

Impressive full body fitness development

For those who want to earn actual results in weight loss / fat loss, full body strength, stamina, mobility and cardiovascular development, this guide encompasses all these aspects of fitness.

Short workouts only

For most trainers wishing to earn meaningful fitness results, the time needed for workouts can be a significant issue. But it's still possible to get the same results with short workouts. We just have to train in a specific way.

No workout equipment needed

If we are not reliant on fitness equipment or gym opening times, we can train anywhere. We don't have to travel to a gym, or even set up gym equipment in our homes. We can choose exactly when and where we want to exercise.

A regular exercise routine with a goal in mind is an invaluable quality of life upgrade for everyone. As a fitness professional with personal training experience over a twenty-five-year period, training others and myself, I fully understand that

How to Use This Book

To use this book, you can simply choose one of the pre-made workout routines, learn the exercises, and start working out. But to get the most out of it, especially if you are a beginner, I would advise to read the whole thing and plan as you read through. If you do this, you'll have a good understanding of why you are doing what you are doing and by the time you finish, you'll have your very own workout routine that aligns with your fitness level and personal goals. You'll also have a better understanding of why this method works.

So if you are already comfortable and confident with this type of training, try out one of the premade exercise routines, then use the blank training cards to make changes if you want to add or switch out any exercise choices. You can do this as many times as you like.

If you are new to exercise or have not trained with quick, intense workouts before, you will have a much better insight into the way this training should work if you read the contents thoroughly before you start working out.

When you are ready to start training, there are three premade routines in "The workouts" section. I would advise starting with the beginner workout to test your fitness level. If this is too easy, try the next and so on. If you find that you are not ready for some of the exercises, at this point, you can start to tailor your own routine.

Pre-made exercise routines are great! But none of us are at exactly the same fitness level. For example, there may be some movements that you can perform perfectly to give yourself a good challenge. These movements might not be suitable for me as I am not yet conditioned enough to perform them, and vice versa.

The pre-made routines in this guide start with a beginner program card and progress to more advanced and intense routines. These were created and set out in this way, not only to highlight a progression path for the beginner, but to also demonstrate the possibilities of varying intensity during a workout. If you are a beginner and start with the beginner exercise card, you may find the exercises don't offer much challenge, so you may want to take it to the next level on your next training day. But I would always advise that if you start a workout and find that it is lacking, you should finish it and reassess for the next session. This way, you have at least completed a full training session.

When stepping up your training level, you do not necessarily need to progress with the next premade routine completely. You may find some exercise choices from the routine at the next level too difficult at this point, but are able to do others. If this happens, switch out the exercise for a similar variation that you can do.

For example, if you struggle to do full "push ups", you could switch this exercise out with "push ups on knees". There are more ideas for creating your own progressive routine later in the book, but I mention this here to highlight the point that the premade routines are there as a guide and starting point for most. With that said, if you find you are able to progress through these as they are set out, great!

The last thing to mention is the exercise choices. I have always been a big advocate of using correct exercise form, so practicing the movements for every exercise we choose to use in our workouts is a big priority in my opinion. Each movement we make is designed to engage certain muscle groups and ranges of movement. If we use bad form or our posture is not right during an exercise, we not only open ourselves up to injury potential, but we miss out on the effect of the exercise or we "dilute the intensity".

There are exercises in this guide that require a "slow and controlled movement". These are great for beginners as they're easier to get to grips with, and help to establish good exercise form practices when compared to explosive movements.

"Explosive" movements play a big part in this guide too. These are designed to use more energy, more muscle groups and therefore tend to be a lot more intense causing us to fatigue more quickly. When we become fatigued, our body and mind will want to make things easier. It's at this point that we really need to concentrate on exercise form as this is where we get the most value from our training.

If you find that part way through a set you become fatigued and struggle to complete repetitions to their full extent, pause, reset your starting position, take a few breaths and perform a single, quality repetition of the exercise, continue this until your set is complete. Often, one good quality repetition of an exercise is better than several bad quality ones.

To help with exercise form, each movement mentioned in the book has an illustration and a written description. The description is set out as step-by-step instructions in a bullet point format style. Follow each bullet point to get the full picture.

Depending on whether you have the paperback or eBook version of this guide, you will also have the option to watch an animated version of each exercise. This may give more clarity and understanding if you need it. There is a QR code associated with each movement for you to scan inside the paperback version and a clickable link to follow in the eBook version.

As mentioned earlier, I highly recommend practicing any exercises that you wish to use in your workouts before you start a full training session.

Health Check

Before you embark on any fitness routine, please consult your doctor or physiotherapist. If you have any health conditions, always check if the type of exercise and exercise choices you intend to involve yourself with.

1. Do not exercise if you are unwell.

2. Stop if you feel pain, and if the pain does not subside, consult your doctor or physiotherapist.

3. Do not exercise if you have taken alcohol or had a large meal in the last few hours.

4. If you are taking medication, please check with your doctor to make sure it is okay for you to exercise.

5. If in doubt at all, please check with your doctor or physiotherapist first – you may even want to take this routine and go through it with them. It may be helpful to ask for a blood pressure, cholesterol and weight check. You can then have these taken again in a few months to see the benefit.

Before you start, commit to at least four weeks of consistent training by making a plan that includes training days, time of training and workout routine you will use (more help with this later in the guide). This will help with initial motivation and focus.

Remember that the opportunity for physical change in our bodies comes from us forcing our bodies to adapt to consistent, challenging exercise, so consistency is key.

Exercise guidelines

For the fitness goal of burning fat and toning muscle, whilst also trying to cut down the time spent exercising, there are a few things we need to consider. Although diet goes hand in hand with exercise choices for any fitness goal, we will not consider it here, as this is a big subject and there are many nuances.

To keep this as simple as possible and to justify the exercise choices and methods in this guide, here is a breakdown of why this type of training fits perfectly with these fitness goals.

Movement

The first point is that body movement uses energy. Using energy is the simplest way for us to tap into our excess fat stores. Continuous, repetitive movement is an excellent way to achieve this whilst also elevating our heart rate and challenging our cardiovascular systems.

Muscle

The second point is that challenging our muscles through their respective range of movements helps to strengthen and tone these muscle groups. This also has a big effect on the fat burning process as muscle needs energy to repair, grow and maintain. So, the more lean muscle we have, the better at fat burning we will be.

Intensity

Of course, there are exercise choices for movement and muscle development that vary to the extreme when it comes to intensity. For example, walking on the spot is a way to add movement and lower body muscular development to an exercise routine, but we could also add "tuck jumps". If we perform each exercise for the same amount of time, the "tuck jump" exercise would be a far superior form of expending energy and challenging or developing muscle function.

To get the most value from a quick workout, the overall intensity of the routine should be high. Meaning that each exercise should challenge us and we should move from each exercise to the next without resting. Also, the individual exercises within the workout should be performed at a continuous pace.

For the purpose of this guide, I have included two types of exercise. I have categorised these as: "controlled" and "explosive". Although these are not technically "industry standard" categorisations, I believe this is a great way to identify the approach and expectations when it comes to performing the movement.

Explosive exercises

I've chosen the term "explosive exercise" because the nature of this exercise choice requires us to load a muscle group and "explode" through a movement. An example of an explosive exercise in this particular fitness book is the tuck jump.

At the starting position, we load the muscles of the lower body:

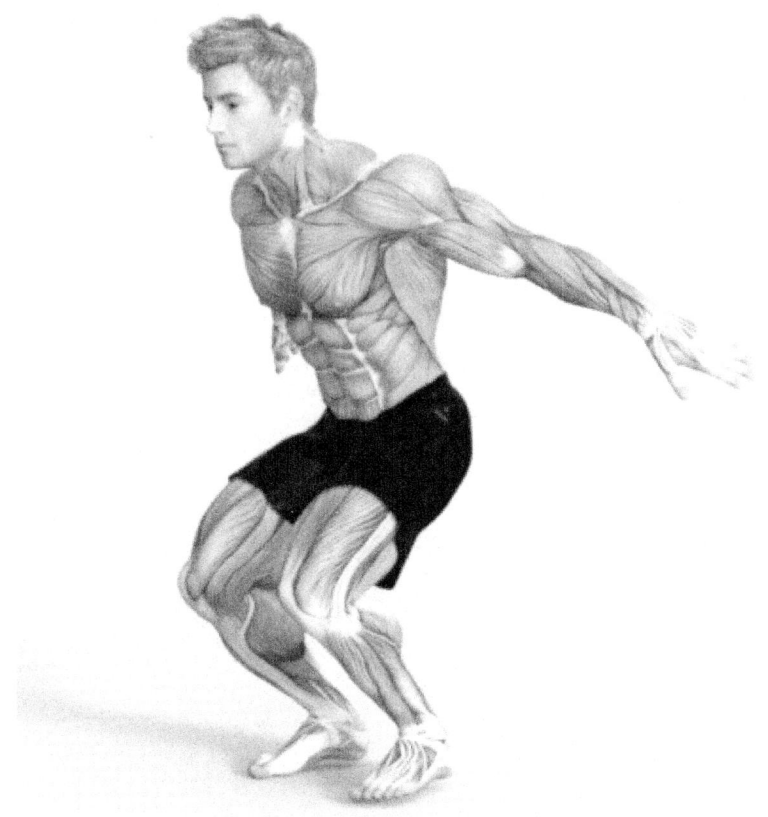

Once in position, we then "explode" through our legs, jumping into the air, whilst bringing our knees to our chest:

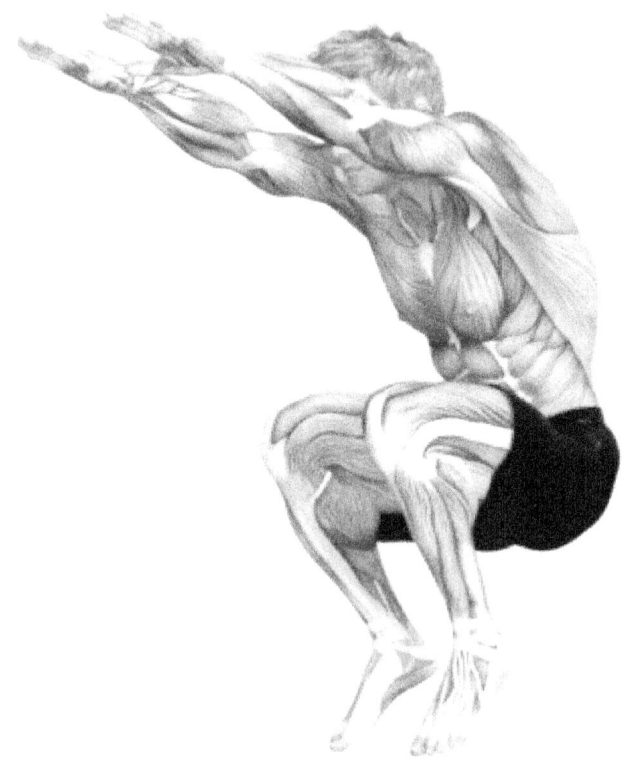

I would classify the tuck jump as a more advanced explosive exercise choice, but it serves as a great example of this type of movement. If this particular movement looks too advanced for your current fitness level, there are other explosive exercises that are more appropriate for beginners or less conditioned trainers.

It's not true for all explosive movements listed in this book, but generally speaking, this type of exercise gives us a certain "loss of control effect" at certain parts of the movement. For instance, as we are at the mercy of gravity, we could not "hold the mid position" if we wanted to.

Controlled exercises

As opposed to explosive exercises, controlled movements are those which we have full control over throughout the repetition. "Push ups on knees" is a beginner friendly example of such an exercise:

During the start position, we load the muscle groups. In this case it's the upper body (chest, shoulders and triceps):

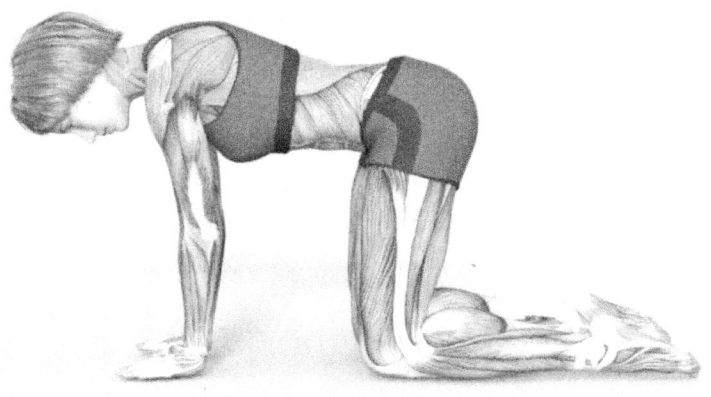

Once in position, we lower our upper body towards the floor:

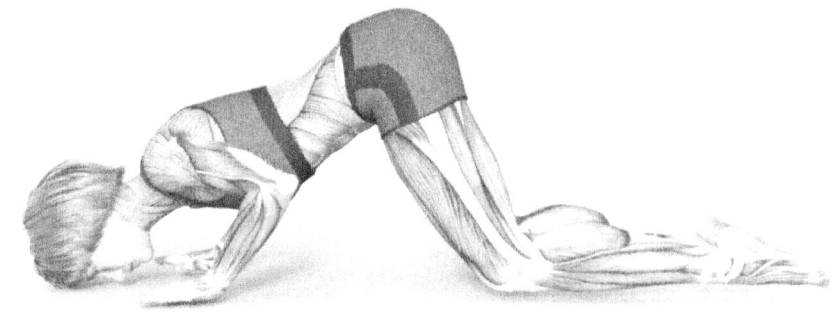

Throughout the transition from the start position to the top of movement, we have full control over the movement: we can hold at any point and we are fully responsible for the speed of the repetition. The speed of the repetition should be continuous and controlled, but not "explosive". I would recommend a full repetition of a controlled exercise to take 4 seconds, 2 seconds to reach the top of movement (Mid way point) and 2 seconds to return to the start position.

It is plausible to use these controlled movements "explosively". But I would consider this an advanced training method, or if the fitness goal was to increase muscle power. For the purpose of this guide and the fitness goal of fat burning and muscle tone, my recommended implementation of the exercise is probably the best fit for most trainers.

Workout length and volume

The volume of a workout is the measure of repetitions and workload in each training session. Or the number of exercise choices and how many times you perform each exercise in each training session. This links the time spent on each training session to the volume of the workout. For effective results with quick workouts, we need to consider the exercise volume whilst keeping the intensity high during training sessions.

When planning our workouts, we should consider several factors:

The time you want to spend on your training session

How much time can you invest in each workout session on a regular basis? I believe it's possible for most people to comfortably find thirty minutes every day for exercise, especially if there is no travelling to a gym or equipment set up involved. This is more than enough time per session to have a fantastic workout using the methods in this guide. We may even need far less time. A ten-minute workout can be extremely intense and challenging depending on the exercise choices we use, but I would suggest the ten-minute mark to be the shortest workout where possible.

The exercise choices you would like to incorporate

The choice of exercises in your workouts will have a big impact on your results. A ten minute daily workout using a single intense exercise such as burpees can be excellent for full body fitness results. If you decide to use the same timeframe of ten minutes and the same volume of training, but instead of using the single exercise of burpees you use arm circles, a far less demanding exercise, the intensity and full body fitness benefits will be extremely different.

Your current fitness level

If you are a beginner to exercise, you may find that more intense exercises such as burpees are far too challenging and you are only able to perform a few repetitions before complete exhaustion, causing your workout to last for a very short time. This is ok as long as you are performing the exercise correctly and you are not overexerting yourself to the point of injury. There are several suggested methods of using quick workouts in this guide and I would advise that if you are new to exercise that you start with the beginner routine at first. By all means, add a more intense exercise to the end of the routine if you feel you are ready.

More advanced or more conditioned trainers have the opportunity to try some of the intense workout methods, such as "Single exercise" routines, as they may have the ability to perform intense exercise choices for a prolonged period, giving them a substantial training session.

The training method you want to use

In the previous chapter, different types of training were highlighted; the tonne, timed, single exercise, and supersets. If you have a planned list of exercises that you wish to use in your workout, you can decide how you run through them. Do you want to run the routine in a superset style, timed routine, or something else? The volume of your workload won't change much, if at all whichever type of method you choose, but the time per exercise session will. For example, a superset routine will have rest periods throughout adding to the overall time it takes to complete the list of exercises, so this is something to consider if you wish to cut down on time spent training and add extra intensity.

So, how long should your workout be? As mentioned, and for the purpose of this guide, I would suggest that you aim for at least ten minutes of the most intense exercise choices that you are capable of. The idea is to challenge your body through a period of sustained movement. If your ability is a single exercise from the beginner routine, great! You have a big scope for progression. At the other end of the scale, if you can perform none stop, more advanced exercises like tuck jumps and burpees, I would suggest that you limit your workouts to no more than thirty minutes.

It may take a few weeks of trial and error in order to find your ideal workout length and volume, but this is all part of the process. During this time, you will be developing your fitness levels, exercise technique and establishing a habit. It may feel a bit clunky at first, but if you stick at it, try a few different methods and exercises, you will find your flow.

Exercise Cards Explained

Exercise cards are a big part of this book, and I've always advised anyone who sets out to achieve meaningful change with fitness to get this in place before starting. Readers of my other guides will probably find this tiresome, but I can't overstate the value that I have found from using a routine card in my own training and that of my clients enough.

A few of the benefits of exercise cards:

- They give us a plan and a goal
- They give us motivation
- They give us accountability
- They give us progress reports
- They help us to identify individual strengths and weaknesses

The exercise cards consist of three parts. Here's an overview of how the cards work and an explanation of each section.

Section 1

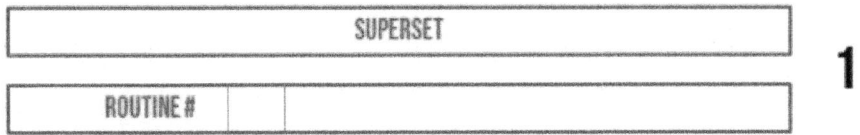

Section 1 has space for the name or type of routine. In the example above, this is called "Supersets". All the pre-made routines in this guide have this filled in already, but if you create your own, you can decide on the name of your workout.

Below the name of the workout, there is a "Routine #" field. I have included this for long-term tracking of fitness progress. This is very useful for those who stay consistent with training and upgrade their routines over time. When an upgrade is made, a new routine is planned, and a new card used, the number here increases. There is also a space next to this for notes or dates.

Section 2

EXERCISE	REPS/ TIME

2

Section 2 is where we input our exercise choices. The first exercise of our routine is listed in the top space and subsequent exercises underneath. We perform the exercises from top to bottom according to the list.

Next to each exercise, in the next column, we have a section to record the amount of repetitions or amount of time we plan to perform each exercise for. This can be pre planned if we are working from a set number of repetitions style workout, or it can be used to record "reasonable failure" (The amount of repetitions we got to before we could not complete any more with good exercise form).

For timed workouts, this should be pre planned and entered before the workout. Depending on the exercise, time spent or repetitions performed on each movement can vary from exercise to exercise.

Section 3

WEEKS	MON	TUE	WED	THURS	FRI	SAT	SUN
1							
2							
3							
4							
5							

3

The third section on each card is an excellent accountability tool. Forward planning of our workout schedule can be entered here for several weeks ahead of time. The left-most column lists the upcoming weeks in ascending order. The top field of the rest of the table shows the days of the week.

We can plan our training sessions for several weeks ahead and specify which days of each week we plan to train on. To do this, we simply mark the appropriate box with a "*". Once we have completed the planned workout, we can check it off. If we miss a planned workout, we can also mark it to signify a missed session.

As mentioned, this is a great planning, motivational and accountability tool. If you are planning on making serious progress with your workouts, this should absolutely be utilised.

Workouts

This section is dedicated to workout, routine examples and exercise descriptions. Starting with a beginner routine and moving through intermediate to advanced, each program card is followed by the exercise descriptions and illustrations associated with the workout.

The routines in this section all follow a simple sets and reps or timed method, meaning they are designed to be completed with a pre-planned range in mind. The "Sets" and "Reps/time" fields have been left blank, as this is very subjective between trainers. This is for you to decide. If you are not sure where to start, I would suggest that each exercise is performed between 1–3 times (sets) using between 10-15 repetitions. If you would prefer to use a timed exercise slot, I'd advise that you use 1 -3 sets of 30 -60 seconds to start with.

Beginner workout

BEGINNER		
ROUTINE #		

EXERCISE	SETS	REPS / TIME
Stationary march		
Push ups on knees		
Arm circles		
Punch it out		
Cross over lunge		
Kickbacks		
Standing side crunch		
Windmill		
Shoulder reach		
Leg swing (front back)		

WEEKS	MON	TUE	WED	THURS	FRI	SAT	SUN
1	*	*		*	*		
2	*	*		*	*		
3	*	*		*	*		
4	*	*		*	*	*	
5	*	*		*	*	*	
6	*	*		*	*	*	

Stationary march

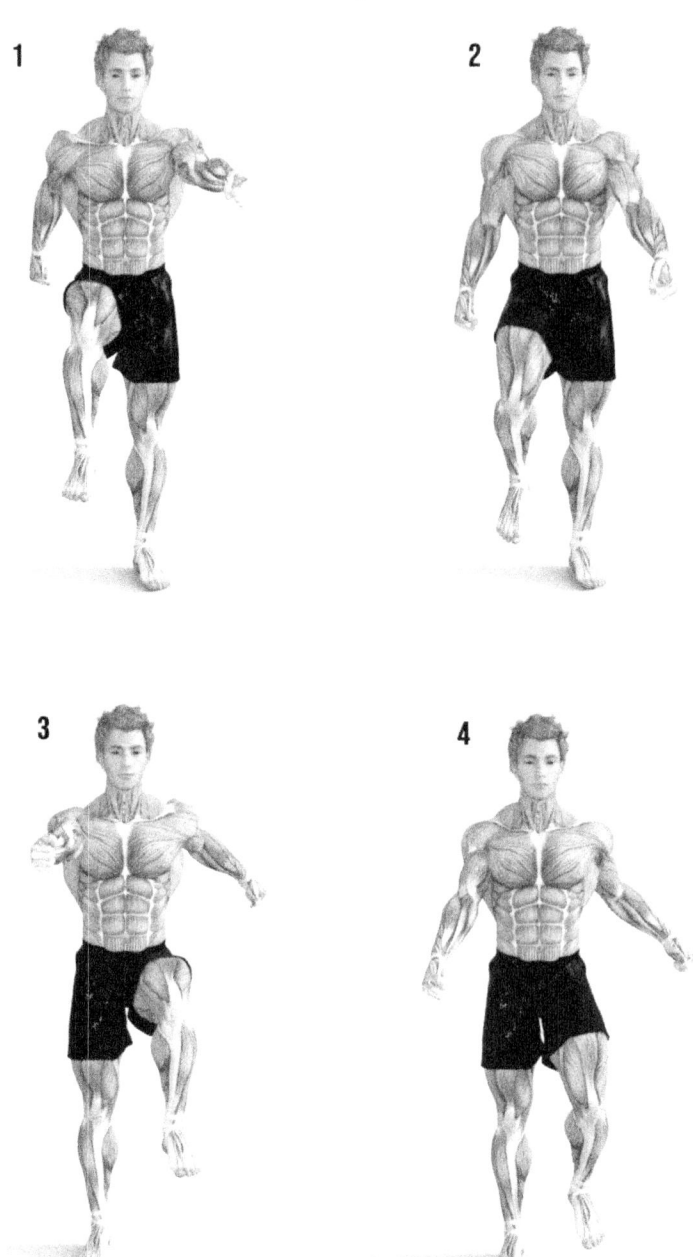

- This is a controlled movement
- From a standing position, lift your right leg so the upper part is parallel to the floor
- As you do this, rotate your left shoulder so your left arm moves to the front of your body
- At the same time, rotate your right shoulder so your right arm moves to the rear of your body
- At the top of this movement, your upper right leg should be parallel with the floor and your left arm should be extended out to your front and parallel, or just above with the floor
- Once this is achieved, return to the start position before immediately mirroring the movement

Arm circles

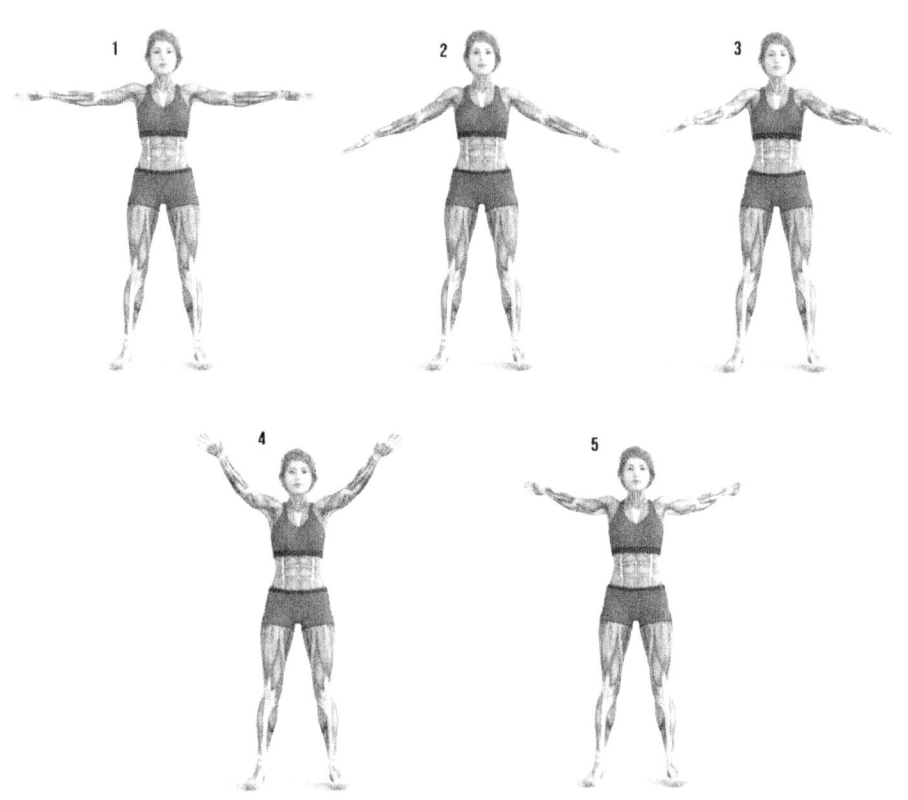

- This is a controlled movement
- Stand with your feet about shoulder width apart and head in a neutral position
- Lift your arms out to your sides so they are fully extended and parallel with the floor
- In a controlled manner, start to rotate your shoulders forward, down, and then back and up
- This should cause your hands to move in circles

During this exercise, it is important to maintain your extended arm position. You may want to vary the range of movement by creating larger circles with your hands. Another variation of this exercise is to perform the exercise by circling the shoulders in the opposite direction.

A common problem area with shoulder mobility is the "upward, rear" movement (Fig 5 on the illustration). If this is difficult for you, slow the movement down at this point and concentrate on the exercise form.

Punch it out (Shadow boxing)

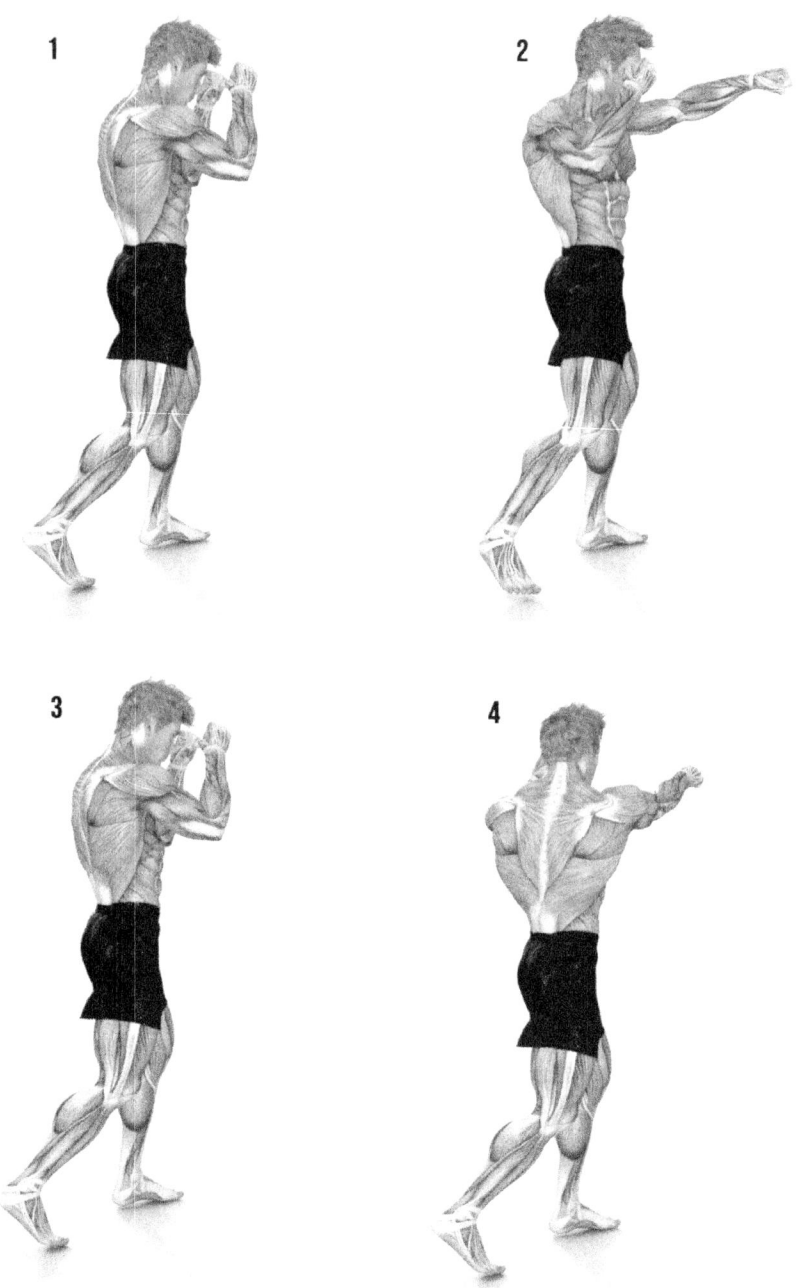

- This is an explosive movement
- Stand with your left foot forward, toes pointing forward and your right foot back, toes pointing slightly to your right
- Distribute your bodyweight evenly between both feet
- Make fists with your hands and lift them so they are in line with the sides of your face and slightly forward
- As you exhale, twist at your waist slightly towards your right-hand side, straighten your left arm to punch. At the top of the movement, your arm should be directly in line with your head, or slightly above and your palm should be facing down
- Once your left hand is back at the starting position, twist at your waist slightly towards your left-hand side and punch forward with your right fist as you did with your left hand

This exercise is based on a traditional boxing stance, but if you wish to change the position of your feet, this is no problem, switching your leading foot from left-to-right mid-way through your exercise set has its benefits and can add variety to this movement.

During this exercise, fatigue can set in, leading to lower punches and a lower "guard position" when returning to the start position before throwing the next punch. Try to be aware of this throughout the set and correct as soon as possible if you need to.

Kickbacks

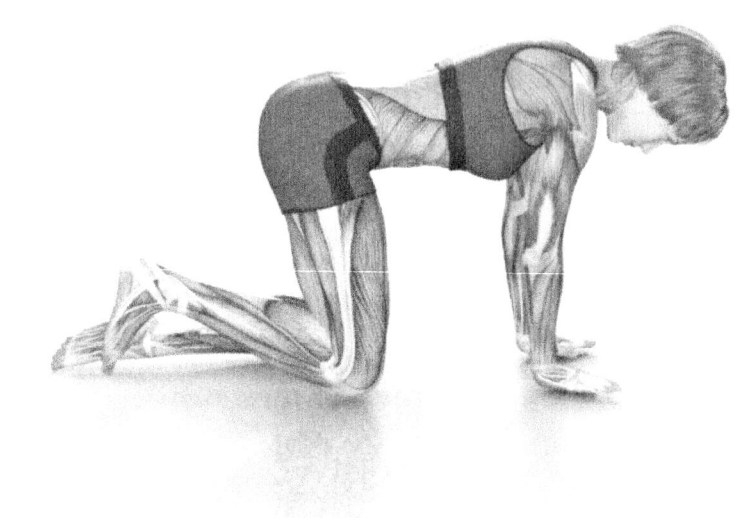

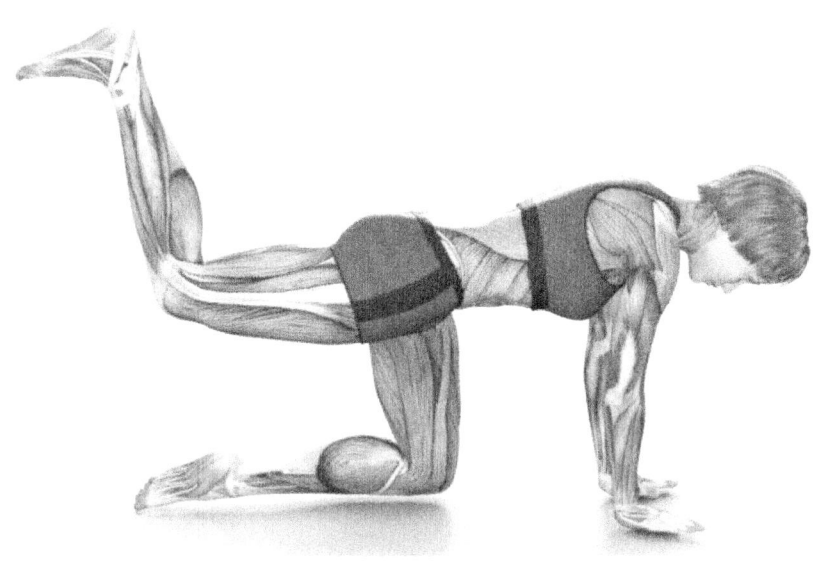

- This is a controlled movement
- Position yourself so that both your knees are in contact with the floor and in line with your hips
- Your shins and tops of your feet should also be in contact with the floor
- Hinge at your hips to bring your upper body forward
- Take the weight of your upper body by placing your hands on the floor so they are in line with your shoulders
- Keep your back flat and maintain this throughout the movement
- Keep your hips and back aligned as you lift your right knee away from the floor slightly by bringing your knee towards your upper body slightly
- Ensure that you transfer your bodyweight evenly between your hands and your left knee
- Once in this position, as you exhale, push your right leg up behind your body
- Once you are at the top of movement, return to the start position as you inhale
- Continue this movement for your planned time slot or planned repetition range, before repeating with the opposite leg

This is an exercise that may look simple, but there are some common pitfalls for some trainers. This is an exercise that targets the glutes (bum / butt). A rotation of the hips during the movement can dilute the effectiveness of the exercise and put a strain on the lower back. This is the most common mistake during this exercise and due to the position, it's hard to check exercise form even with the use of a mirror.

If you use this exercise, this is something to be aware of. Keep your hips in line with your upper body throughout the movement, even if it feels as if the range of movement restricts you. You should feel more effect on your glutes with this in mind.

Standing side crunches

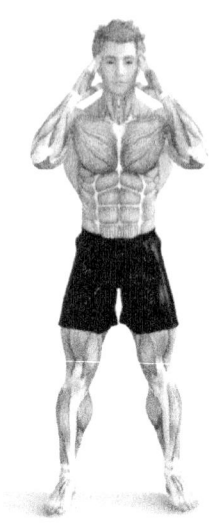

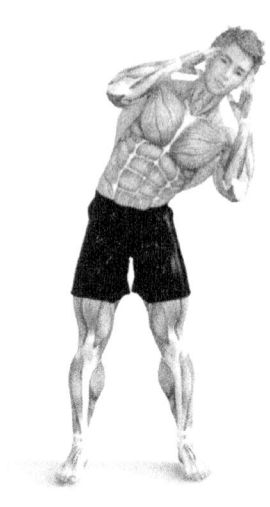

- This is a controlled movement
- Stand with your feet about shoulder width apart
- Place your fingers on the sides of your head by bringing your arms out to your sides and bending your elbows
- As you exhale tilt your upper body to your left hand side ensuring that you maintain a neutral sagittal plan (forward / backward movement)
- Both feet should remain firmly planted on the floor
- Once you reach the top of movement, inhale and return to the start position
- Once you have completed your planned workload on one side, repeat on the opposite side

This is a slow and controlled movement. Always be aware of the "front / back movement" of your upper body. We are aiming to keep this neutral; it's easy to lose awareness of this during the exercise.

Although the description states that this should be performed on one side at a time, it is plausible to alternate, meaning a movement to your left side, followed by a movement to your right side. If you wish to perform the exercise this way, I'd advise a clear pause or "reset" at the start position before each alternate side movement. This way, you will be more focused on the exercise form.

Windmill

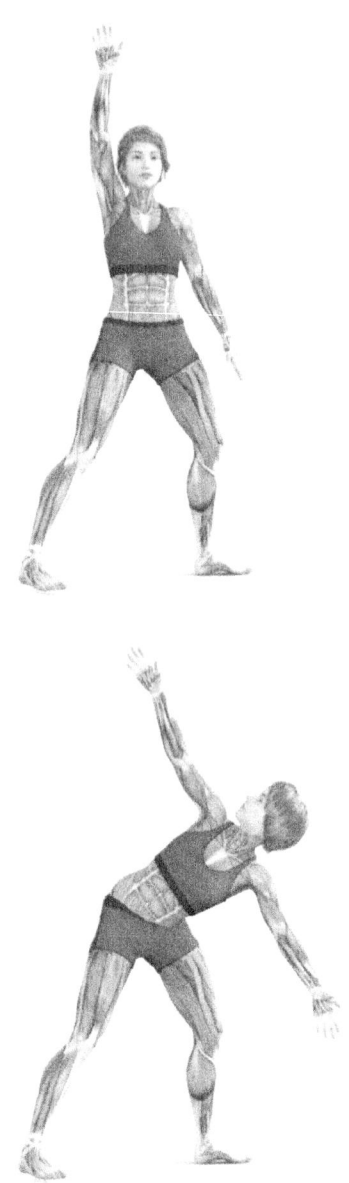

- This is a controlled movement
- Stand with your feet flat on the floor about so they are further than shoulder width apart
- Twist your ankles so your toes point more towards your left hand side
- Reach directly above your head with your extended right arm
- As you exhale, hinge at your hips to drop your upper body towards your left hand side
- As you move, extend your left arm and up along the mid line of your body
- Continue until you feel the stretch in your upper glute/ lower back on your right hand side
- Once at the top of the movement, inhale and return to the start position.
- Complete the workload in this direction before repeating in the opposite direction

This is a controlled stretch and strengthening exercise that's often used for the lower back and posterior chain. Be aware that this can be a tricky exercise for the beginner, so if you are starting out with this and are unsure, test your range of movement.

If you can continue the movement until the hand of your leaning side touches the floor, this is the maximum range of the exercise and is the target we should aim for. But for many, this exercise requires some conditioning before this is achieved.

Leg swing (front back)

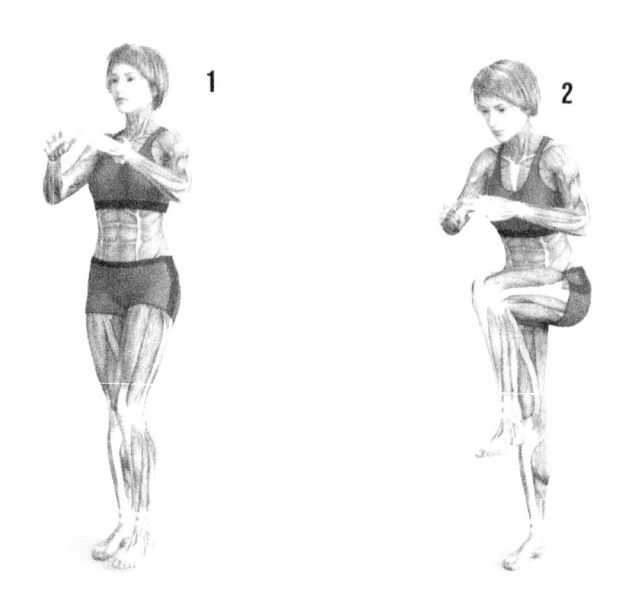

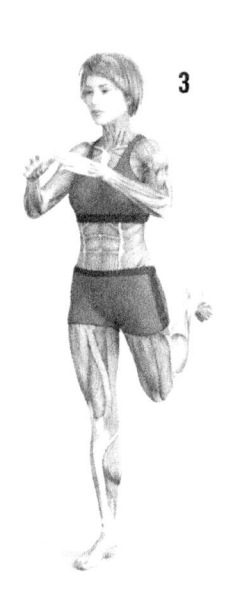

- This is a controlled movement
- Stand straight with your feet about hip width apart and bring your hands up towards the front of your upper body. This is for balance
- Shift your bodyweight to your right foot before lifting your left foot off the floor. Bend the knee and lift your left leg upwards slightly to do this
- Once you have your balance in this position, continue the upward movement of your left leg by bringing the knee towards your upper body
- Once at your maximum range, drop your left leg again moving through the start position to extend to your rear
- Once at your maximum range of movement, repeat the previous two steps continuously until you have completed your planned workload and repeat on the opposite leg

When performing this exercise, you should ensure that your hips stay in line with your upper body to get the most concentrated effect on the working muscle groups. During the forward movement of the leg, it is possible to add a small abdominal crunch at the top of the movement. This will enhance the exercise, but I would advise that this is only performed by those who are confident with the other parts of the movement.

Intermediate workout

INTERMEDIATE		
ROUTINE #		

EXERCISE	SETS	REPS / TIME
Rope less jump		
Prone shoulder tap		
Alternating lunge		
Stationary march		
Uppercut march		
Jumping jacks		
Alternate knee to elbow		
Alternate squat thrust		
Toe touches		
Squat & calf raise		

WEEKS	MON	TUE	WED	THURS	FRI	SAT	SUN
1	*	*		*	*		
2	*	*		*	*		
3	*	*		*	*		
4	*	*		*	*	*	
5	*	*		*	*	*	
6	*	*		*	*	*	

Ropeless jump rope

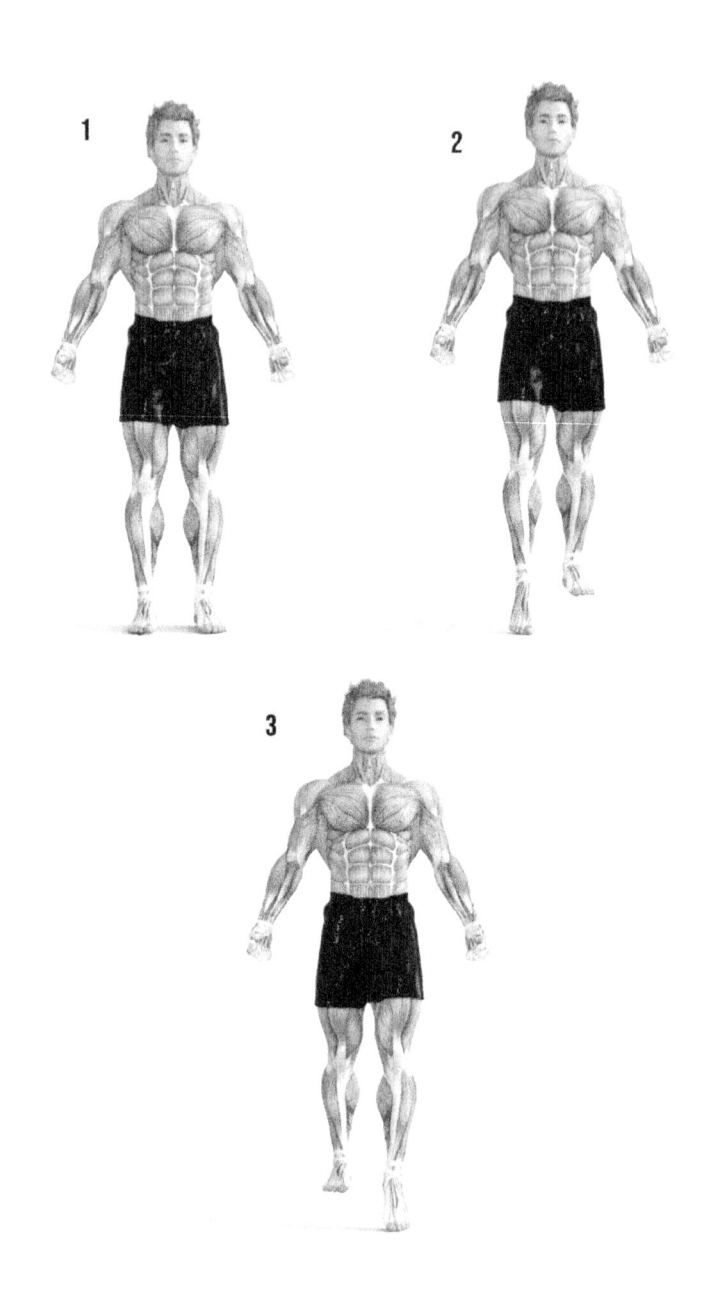

- This is an explosive movement
- Stand with your feet about hip width apart and toes facing forward
- Your arms should be run level with your midline and out to your sides slightly, hands made into fists and palms facing forward
- As you throw an imaginary skipping rope from your back, over your head and towards your toes, shift your body weight to your left foot so your right foot lifts off the ground slightly
- With your right toes just off the ground and your body weight fully transferred to your left foot, use the front of your left foot to push off the ground to perform a low "hop
- As soon as you land, perform the same movement, but switch feet so your right foot becomes the foot that performs the hopping movement

The main reason for using a rope less skipping exercise is to keep the movement continuous. If the trainer is not proficient at using a skipping rope, there will be a lot of time spent stopping to reset the rope when it gets caught, so this dilute the intensity of the exercise. But if you have a rope and have mastered a continuous flow, definitely use it for this exercise.

If you are struggling to get the flow with this exercise, try hopping on one foot, whilst toe tapping the floor with the opposite toes for three to five repetitions before switching to the other for another three to five.

The skipping pattern shown here is known by some as "boxer style" or "the boxer skip". This is because it's commonly used in boxing training for fat burning, endurance in the lower legs and to develop agility. If you want to step up the intensity of this exercise, you can switch to jumping with both feet at the same time. If you do this, keep your body weight distributed evenly between both feet.

Prone shoulder tap (Controlled)

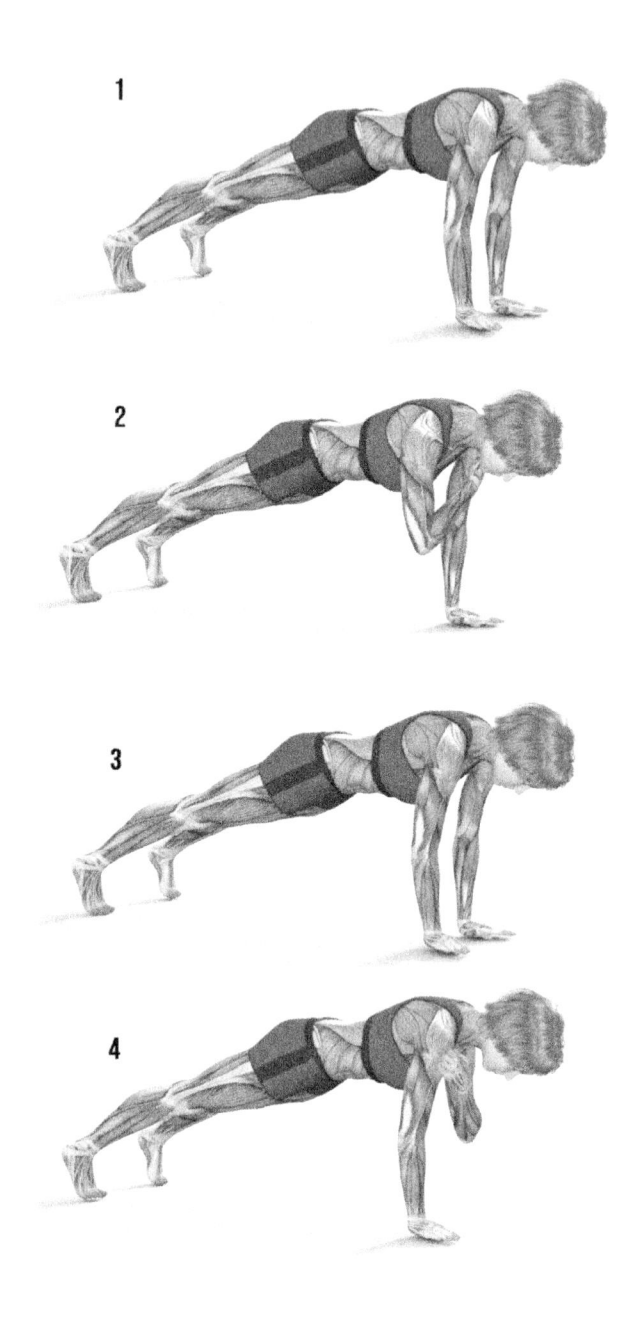

1

2

3

4

- This is a controlled movement
- Assume a push up position; Palms on the floor in line with the fronts of your shoulders, arms straight with a slight bend in the elbows, legs straight and toes in contact with the floor. Keep your back flat and head in a neutral position
- As you exhale, shift your upper body weight so it runs through your left palm
- Once you are stable, in a controlled manner, lift your right hand away from the floor by bending at the elbow and reach across your upper body to tap your left shoulder
- After your palm makes contact with tour shoulder, in the same controlled manner, return it to the start position
- Once back at the start position, repeat the process with your left hand by tapping your right shoulder
- Keep your back flat and abdominals engaged throughout the movement

Although this exercise may look like it's about upper body strength alone, there is actually a big focus on the development of abdominal and core strength involved, too. Engaging your abdominals and making sure your back does not arch or sag throughout this movement can be more challenging than the shoulder tap for some, so be aware of this.

If you would like to do this exercise but find that holding the position is too much, you can perform the same exercise but on your knees instead. Simply use the same start position as the "push ups on knees" exercise. If, on the other hand you would like to take this exercise to the next level, you could try holding the tap on your shoulder for a few seconds before returning it to the start position.

Alternating lunge (Controlled)

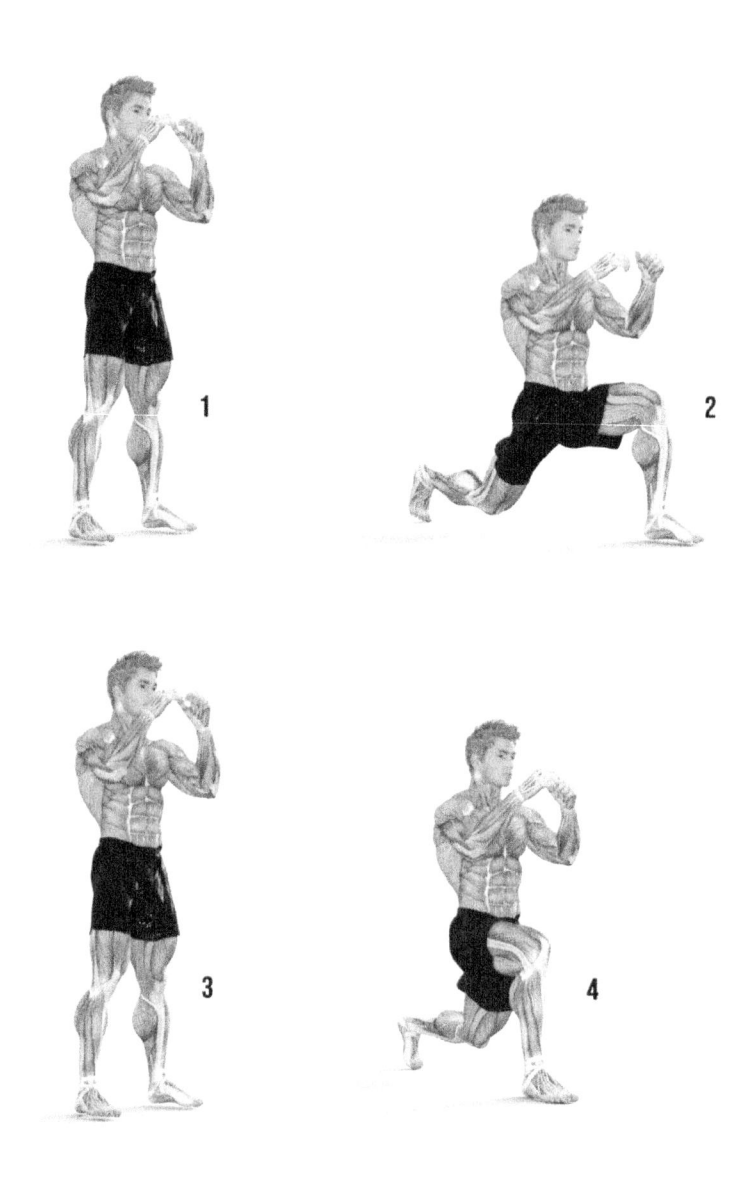

- This is a controlled movement
- Stand with your feet about hip width apart, toes pointed forward and arms lifted out to your front or sides for balance
- Take a stride forward with your left leg
- Lower your body towards the floor by bending the knee of your left leg until your right knee is just about to make contact with the floor
- A right angle should be achieved between the top and the bottom of your leading leg at its rear
- Keep the toes of your trailing leg planted firmly on the floor
- As you exhale, return to the start position and repeat on the opposite leg

Performing this exercise correctly can take some practice. Learning to estimate your stride length in order to form the right angle at the back of your leading leg can take a bit of trial and error. This is important as if your leading knee is in front or backwards of your leading toes when lunging, it can cause undue strain on the knee joint. We should always aim to have our leading knee directly above the mid part of our leading foot. It's worth taking the time to setting up markers on the floor if you are finding this difficult.

An alternative way to perform this exercise is to start at the top of movement (the point that the lunge is performed) and complete a full set on this leg before switching to match on the opposite leg. This way, we take away the guess work when it comes to stride length.

Uppercut march (Explosive)

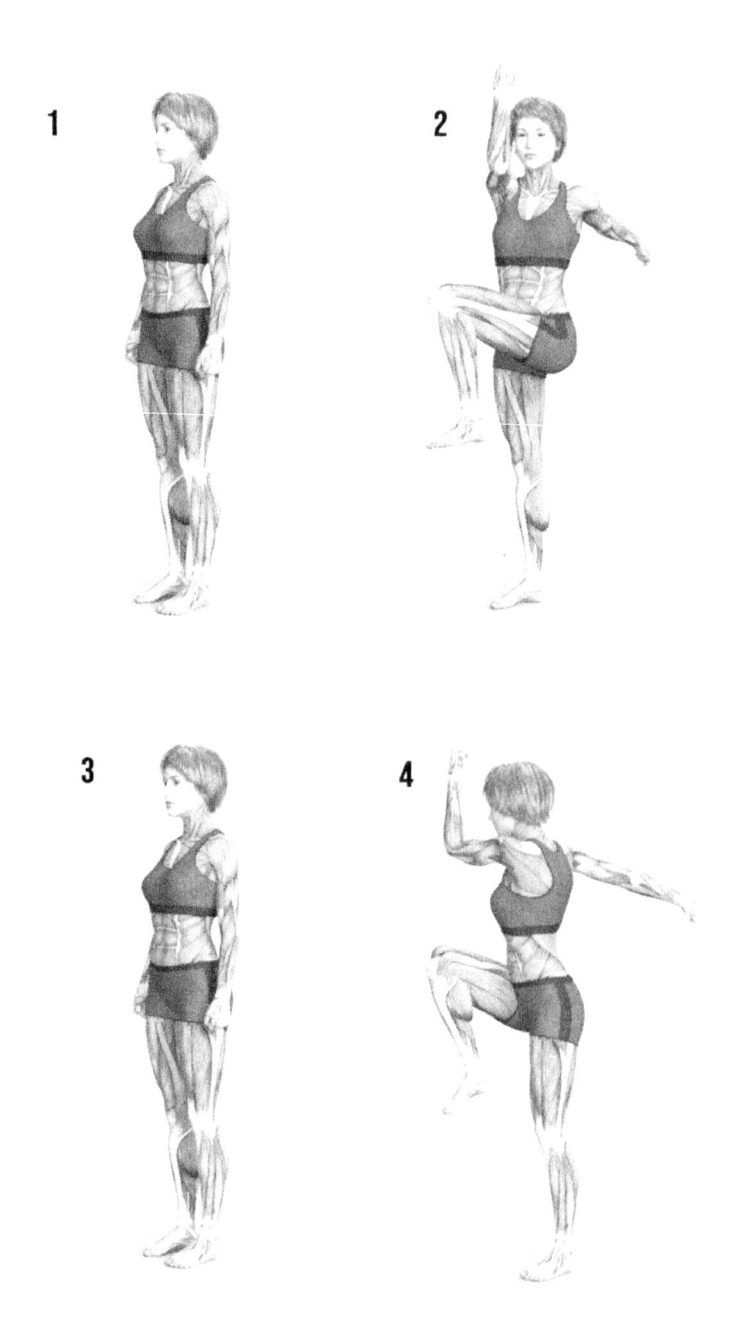

- This is an explosive movement
- Stand with your feet about hip width apart, arms straight by your sides and make fists with your hands. Your palms should start facing towards your body's midline
- As you exhale, shift your bodyweight onto your right foot and lift your left leg until the upper leg is at least parallel with the floor. Bend your knee as you do this
- While you are lifting your left leg, twist at your waist slightly as you lift your right arm up and across your body. Bend your right arm at the elbow and twist your fist so the palm of your right hand finishes above head height and facing towards your rear
- As you perform the previous step, send your straight left arm back towards your rear
- Once you have reached the top of movement, repeat in the opposite direction

This exercise is an explosive movement based on the fact that it simulates a "martial art" move. As it is possible to perform this exercise without losing any control, we can also use it as a controlled movement. In fact, if you are a beginner, this would be a good idea in order to get used to the movement. The exercise requires a lot of muscle groups and a bit of coordination. But once you get the flow, it will be a fantastic explosive exercise to add into your workout that includes good core strength focus as well as balance and strength development opportunities throughout the body.

Alternate knee to elbow (Standing)

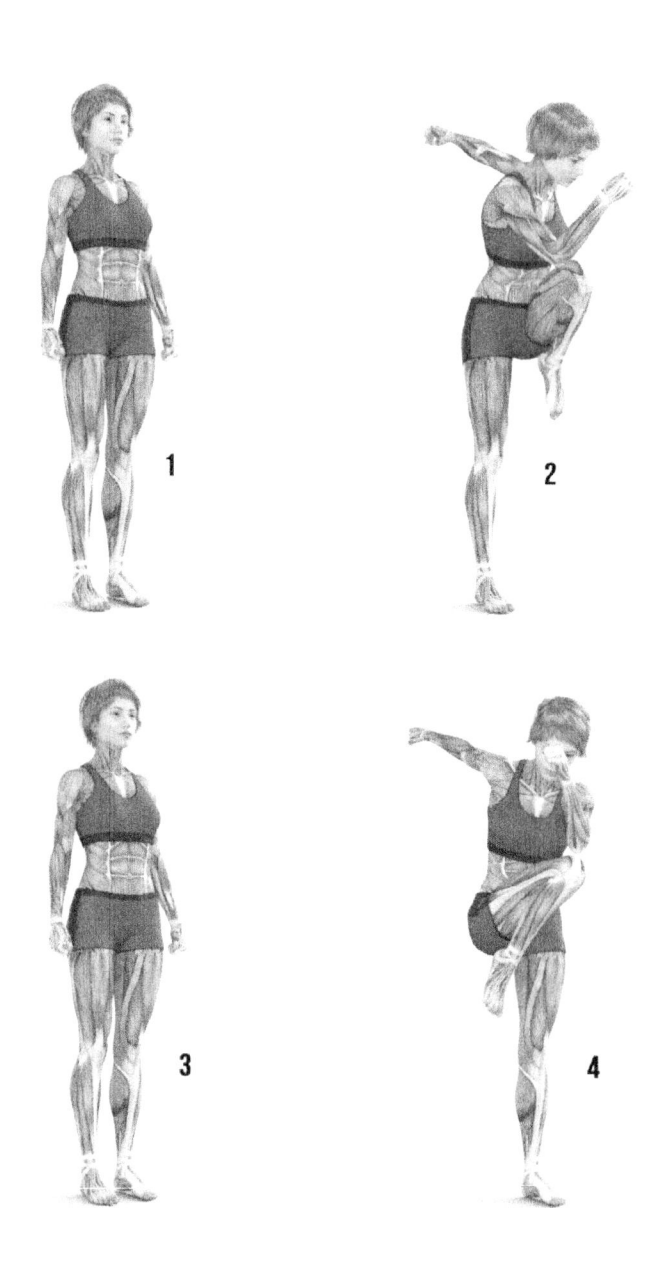

- This is a controlled movement
- Stand with your feet about hip width apart, back flat and head in a neutral position. Arms should be straight and by your sides
- Shift your bodyweight to your right leg and as you exhale, lift your left knee towards your chest. Bend at your left knee as you do this
- As your left knee is lifting towards your chest, being the elbow of your right arm across your body to meet it. Twist slightly at your waist and crunch your abdominals forward slightly
- As your right arm is moving across your body and your left knee is lifting, push your left arm to your rear, keeping it straight
- Once your left knee and right elbow make contact, hold for a brief pause before returning to the start position and repeating in the opposite direction

I decided to label this as a controlled movement as it does require some coordination and the pause at the top of movement gives us great benefits for strength and stability development. This movement can, however, be used as an explosive movement, but I would suggest that if you wish to use it as such, you should become comfortable with the controlled version first.

I would also advise when using this as an explosive movement that the pause at the top of movement and a full reset to the start position is still used. If we get into a fast flow of this exercise, it's easy to dilute the movement by not using its full range.

Another point on this exercise to be aware of is the "elbow to knee contact". If you feel that you can lift your knee higher or crunch your abdominals further forward for extra range of movement, you can lift your knee higher and drop your elbow lower by running your elbow down the inside of your lifted leg, below the knee. This is an excellent way to progress with the movement.

Alternate squat thrust

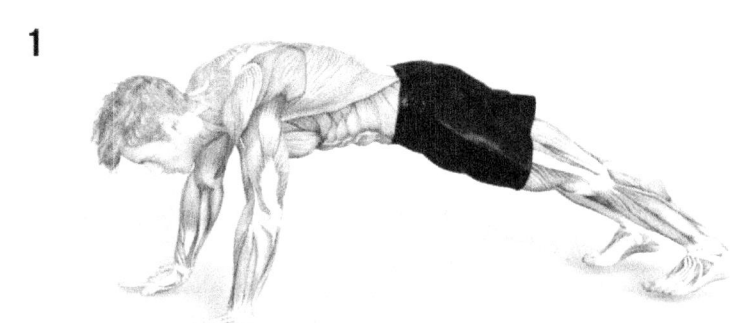

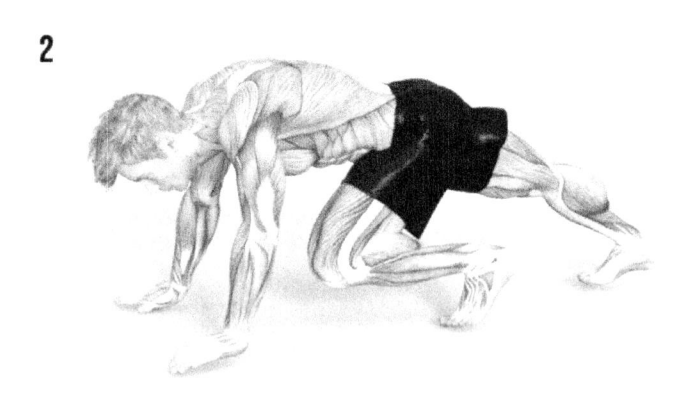

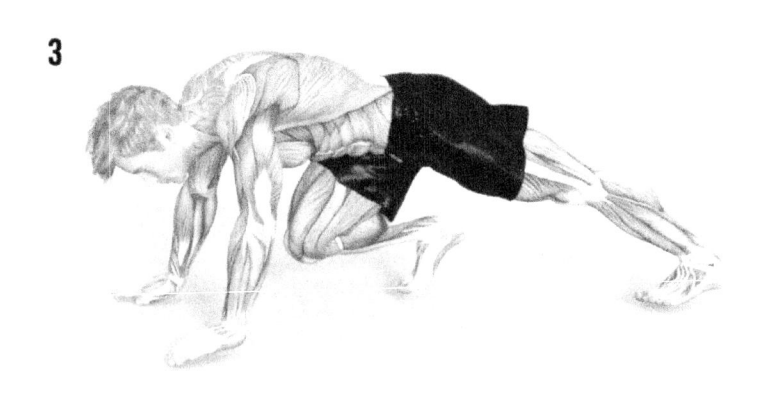

1

2

3

- This is an explosive movement
- Position yourself as you would in order to perform a full push up. Palms on the floor, about shoulder width apart, back flat and toes firmly planted on the floor
- As you exhale, push your left knee towards your chest by bending at the knee. Ensure you keep the toes of your right foot planted firmly on the floor and your back flat
- Once in this position, immediately return your left leg to the start position as you are bringing your right leg towards your chest
- Continue this pattern until your set is complete

In order to achieve the best results, the cadence of this exercise is important. We should perform it continuously. A good guide in regards to the speed is to aim to be bringing one of your knees towards your chest every second in an alternate pattern.

Fatigue in the shoulders is common on this exercise for those who are not used to full push ups, but the more time spent performing squat thrusts, the less this will be an issue as the muscle groups responsible for holding the upper body in this position will be suitably challenged.

During this exercise, be aware of your back position. Ideally, your back should stay flat throughout the movement, meaning that it should not tilt from side to side and it should not become rounded.

Toe touches (Controlled)

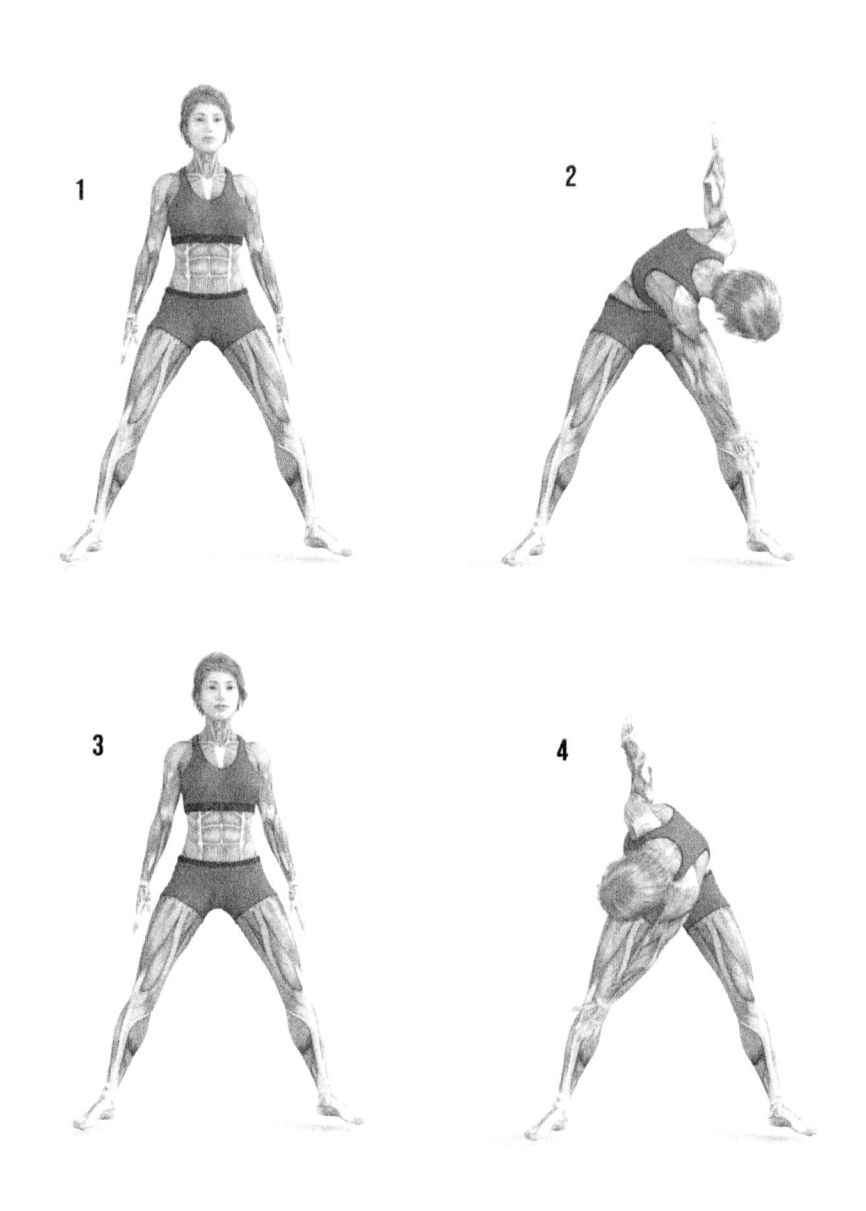

1

2

3

4

- This is a controlled movement
- Stand straight. Back flat, head in a neutral position and arms by your sides
- Your feet should be flat on the floor and firmly planted with a spacing that's past shoulder width. Toes should be pointed at slight angles away from your midline
- As you exhale, hinge forward at your hips and twist from your lower abdominals towards your left hand side. With your right hand, reach towards your left toes
- Push your left arm towards your rear to help with balance and rotation
- ** Once you have reached your maximum range of movement, and feel you can increase the stretch, slowly increase the curve of your spine from bottom to top
- Your legs should stay straight, with a slight bend in the knees and feet should be firmly planted on the floor throughout the movement
- Once you have reached your full range of movement, hold for several seconds before reversing the movement to return you to the start position, then repeat in the opposite direction

This exercise should be performed in a slow and controlled manner. The range of movement for toe touches can vary dramatically from trainer to trainer, so it's really important that you approach this exercise with care. If you can feel the stretch along your hamstrings by only achieving a small movement, this is your specific working range. The more you perform this exercise, the bigger your range of movement will become; you may even find this happens from repetition to repetition.

** I consider increasing the stretch by rounding the spine a fairly advanced move as this does require control and spinal awareness. If you are new to this and wish to try it, you can practice a "spinal roll down". Practice the spinal roll down to get a better idea of how to increase the range of movement with this exercise.

- Start by standing or sitting with a flat back and head in a neutral position
- Tilt your chin down slowly until it touches your neck. This is the mobility of your upper spine
- From this position, move your head forward and down to mobilise your upper/ mid-section of your spine (between your shoulder blades

- From this position, start to perform a crunch with your upper abdominals mobilising your mid / lower spine
- From this position, perform a crunch with your lower abdominals to mobilise your lower spine
- Reverse this process in a controlled manner until you reach the start position again

Squat and calf raise (Controlled)

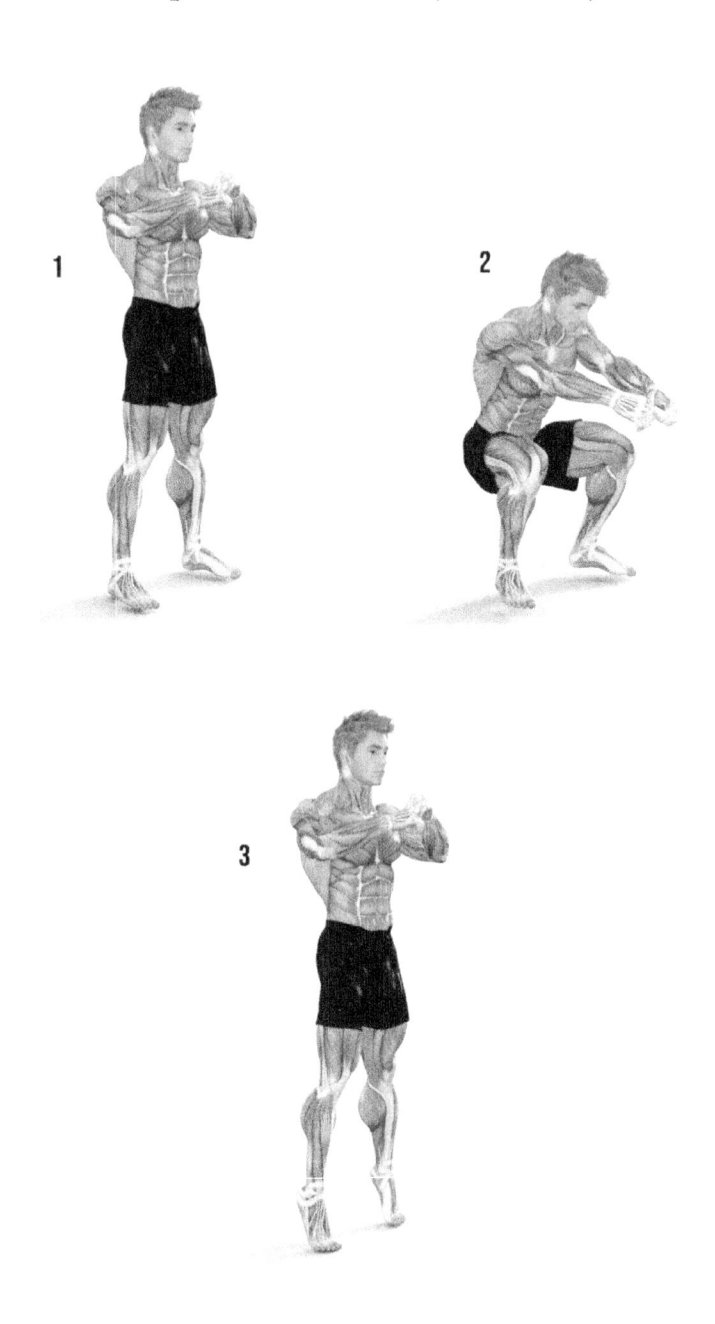

1

2

3

- This is a controlled movement
- Stand with a flat back and feet about shoulder width apart, toes slightly turned out
- Lift your arms to your front or out to your sides for balance
- As you inhale, bend at your knees to lower your upper body towards the floor
- Ensure your feet stay firmly planted and avoid lifting your heels. You should lower until your upper legs are parallel with the floor
- Once at the top of this movement, exhale and push through the centre of your feet as you straighten your legs, returning you to the start position
- Once back at the start position, shift your bodyweight onto the front of your feet and lift your heels away from the floor until your full bodyweight is distributed evenly through your toes on both feet
- Once at the top of this movement, return to the start position

This is a double movement that targets your upper leg muscles during the squat and your lower leg muscles during the calf raise. Most trainers find it more helpful to have their arms positioned across their upper body for balance, but it's also ok to have them out to your sides. This is personal preference.

When performing the second part of this exercise, you can pause and bring your feet closer together for the calf raise if you wish. This may give you a more intense calf raise. If you wish to try this, remember to reset your stance for the squat, ready for the next repetition.

Perform this exercise with a "2 second lower" into the squat and a "2 second return" and the same with the calf raise, so each repetition should take 8 seconds in total.

Advanced workout

ADVANCED		
ROUTINE #		
EXERCISE	SETS	REPS / TIME
Tuck jumps		
Push-ups Knee to elbow		
High kicks		
Power push-ups		
Speed skater		
Squat jacks		
Burpees		
Squat thrust		
Hand walks		

WEEKS	MON	TUE	WED	THURS	FRI	SAT	SUN
1	*	*		*	*		
2	*	*		*	*		
3	*	*		*	*		
4	*	*		*	*	*	
5	*	*		*	*	*	
6	*	*		*	*	*	

Push-ups – Knee to elbow (Controlled)

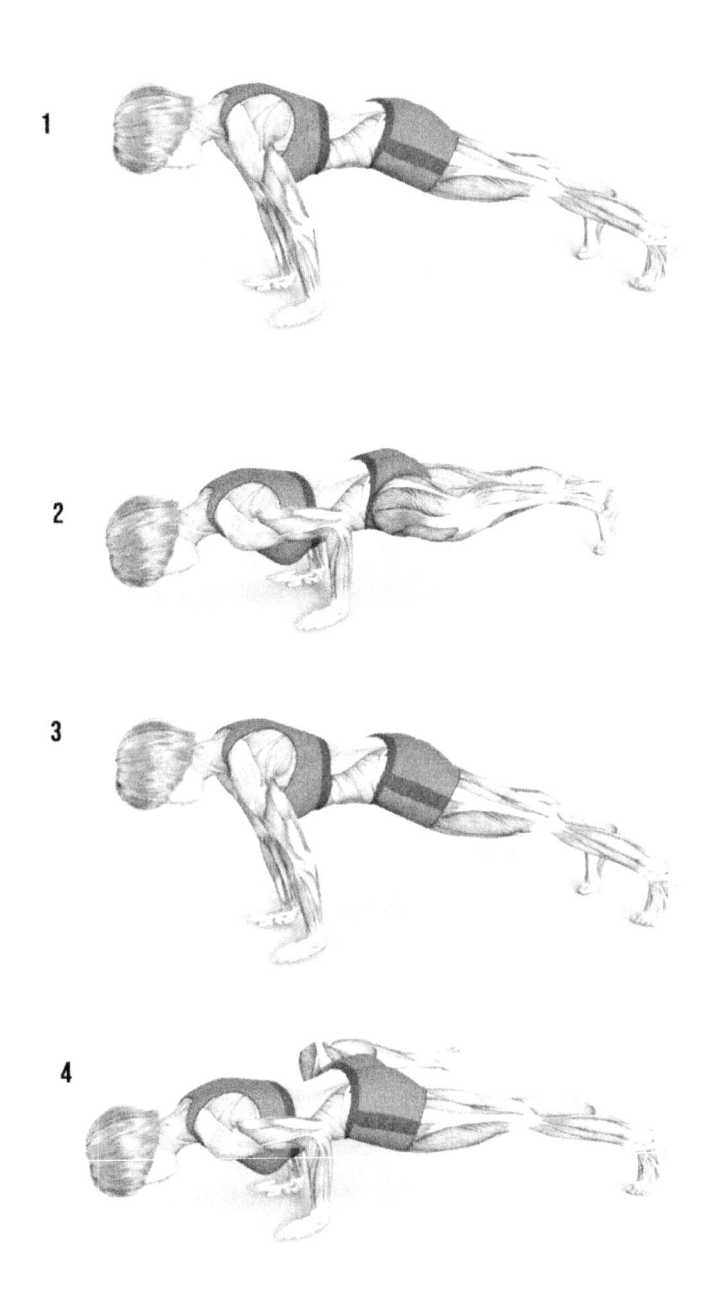

- This is a controlled movement
- Position yourself as if you were about to perform a full push up. Palms on the floor spaced about shoulder width apart and in line with your mid chest, toes firmly in contact with the floor and back flat
- Bend your elbows to bring your upper body towards the floor
- Once your upper arm is about parallel to the floor, pause and shift your lower bodyweight onto your right foot to allow you to lift your left foot away
- Bring your left knee towards your left elbow by bending at the knee and twisting your upper leg
- Once your left knee reaches its maximum range in this direction, return your left leg to the start position
- Once your left leg is firmly planted on the floor again, complete the push up and repeat the process with your right leg

When performing this exercise, ensure that your back remains flat throughout the movement. It should not arch either upwards or downwards and should not tilt from side to side. When bringing the knee to meet the elbow, it can be common to tilt the back towards the opposite side. This movement dilutes the stability benefits that are gained from this exercise where the lower back is concerned, and it can also lead to lower back injury. So keeping the back stable during this movement should be a priority.

If you find that you have less movement with hip rotation and top of movement knee placement than you would like, stay consistent with the exercise and try to increase the range slightly in each session. It also helps with progression for exercises like this. If you slow the exercise down, concentrate on the movement rather than the amount or repetitions and hold at the point that you feel is your maximum range of movement briefly on each repetition.

High kicks - (Explosive)

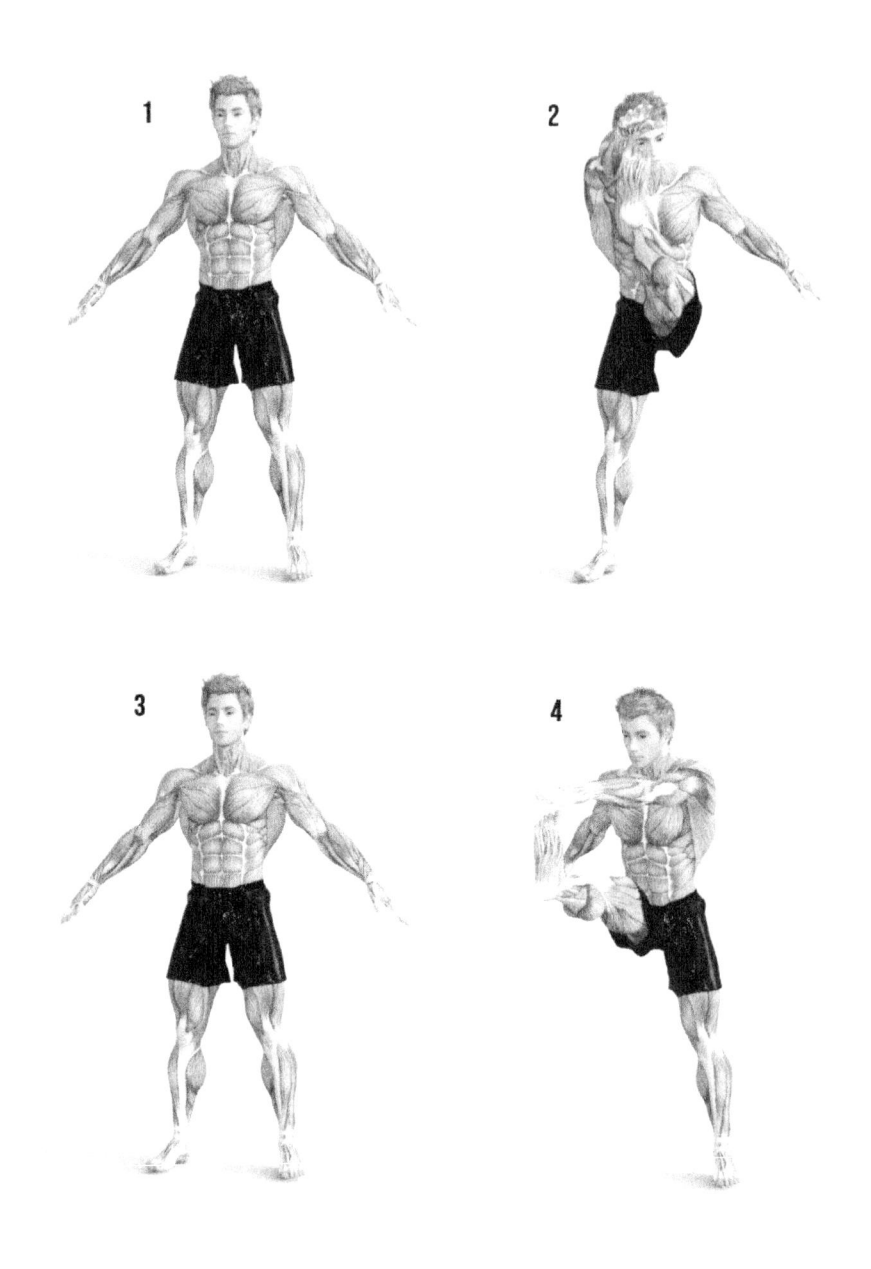

1

2

3

4

- This is an explosive movement
- Stand straight with your feet about shoulder width apart and arms extended and slightly out to your sides. Your knees should have a slight bend in them
- Shift your bodyweight onto your right foot so you are able to lift your left without losing balance
- As you exhale, keeping your leg straight, lift your left leg up in a swift kicking motion
- As your left leg lifts, twist slightly at the hips and perform a shallow crunch with your abdominals to move your torso slightly forward and to your left side
- While your left leg is moving upwards, bring your right arm across your body, as if you were trying to touch your toes to your palm
- Keep your left arm out to your side for balance
- Once at the top of the movement, your leg will naturally begin to fall towards the start position. At this point, take control as you return to the start position
- Reset and perform in the opposite direction

Most of this exercise is controllable, but as we are aiming to perform a high kick, there will be a point for most near the top of movement where the lifted leg is hard to control. Be aware of this and take control of the returning leg as soon as you can. When the foot of the lifted leg makes contact with the floor, you should have full control.

When starting out with this exercise, be aware of the waist twist and abdominal crunch. Ensure your abdominals are engaged and you are aware of the extent of the movement, both in the waist and at the height of your kick. You should perform this exercise with care if you are unfamiliar with the mechanics. Try slow movements with shallow kicks at first to gauge your limits.

Power pushups (Explosive)

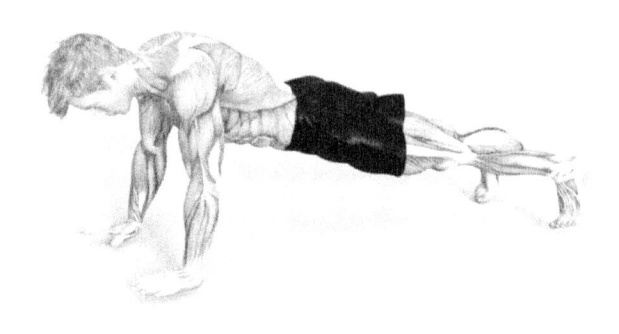

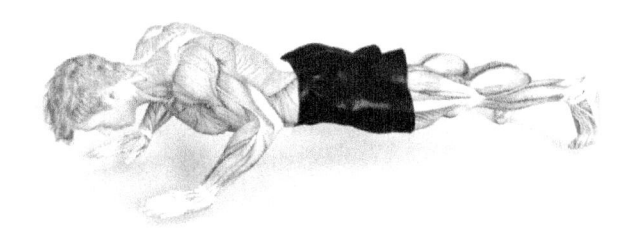

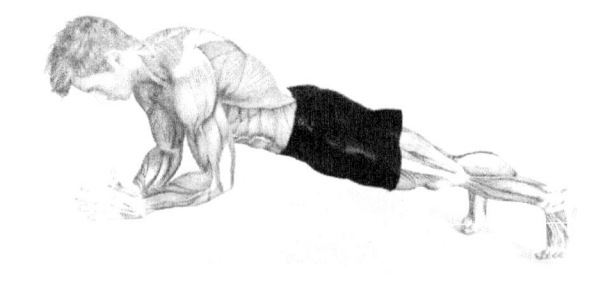

1

2

3

- This is an explosive movement
- Position yourself as if you would when performing full push ups. Palms flat on the floor in line with your mid chest and spaced about shoulder width apart. Your back should be flat and toes firmly planted on the floor
- As you inhale, slowly lower your upper body towards the floor by bending at the elbows. Your elbows should stay close to your sides, but a natural flare outwards is ok
- Once you have lowered your upper body to the point where you feel the stretch across your chest, as you exhale, drive through your palms with enough force to push your upper body away from the floor
- While you are ascending, clap your hands together before returning them to the start position to break your fall.
- As soon as your hands make contact with the floor, continue the downward momentum under control to absorb the shock. This should place you in Figure "2" on the illustration. You will be ready to perform another rep

This is an advanced movement that requires a solid foundation in the muscle groups used to perform push ups. Good shoulder, arm, chest, and back strength should be developed before attempting this exercise.

It's important that you keep a flat back throughout this movement. This is common practice for most exercises like this in order to avoid injury; but in this case, it will also help to keep the benefits of the movement at maximum effect.

Speed skater (Explosive)

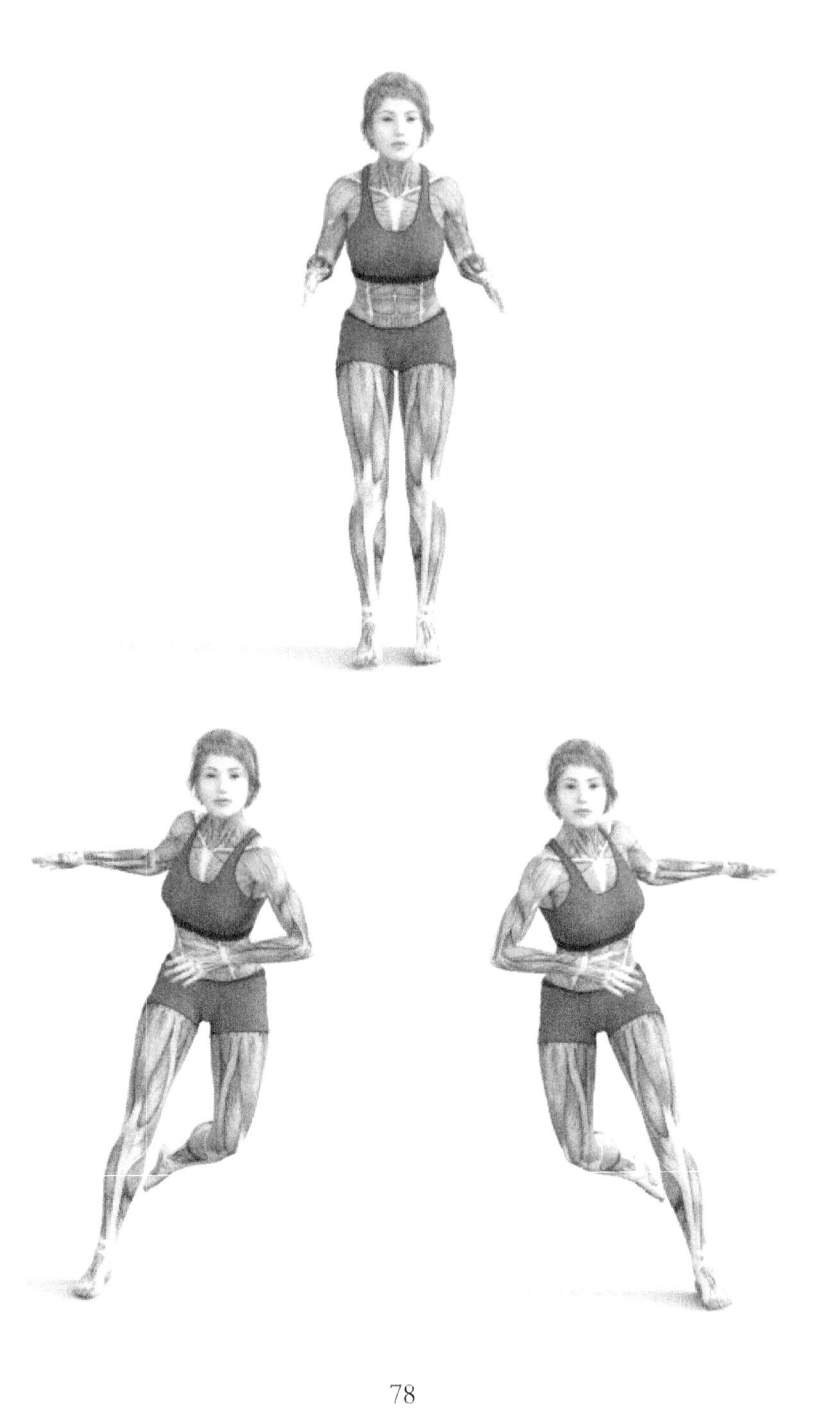

- This is an explosive movement
- Stand with your feet about hip width apart with a slight bend in your knees
- Bend your arms at the elbows to bring your lower arms slightly to your front
- Hinge at the hips slightly to bring your upper body forward. At this point, you should have a lower centre of gravity and be stable on your feet
- Shift your bodyweight onto your right foot and take a small hop to your right from this foot
- As you hop to your right, twist at the waist so that your left shoulder drops slightly in the direction of your right knee
- Your left leg should follow the direction of this movement but remain suspended behind you as a counter balance
- When your right foot is planted on the ground, push off to send your body sideways by bending your knee and prepare to land on your left foot
- As you do this, twist through your waist, this time in the opposite direction to send your right shoulder above your left knee
- Your right leg should now remain suspended behind you and your full bodyweight should be running through your left foot on landing

This exercise takes a lot of coordination and a bit of practice to perfect for most, but it is an excellent movement to add to your workouts for fat burning, balance and power development. When started, the movement should be flowing and continuous and, in most cases, grasping the movement, clicks pretty quickly.

If you would like to slow this down to get used to it, you can perform the movement in one direction and pause before moving in the opposite direction. If you do this, try to pause balancing on one foot with your other leg behind you for balance and your opposite shoulder over the knee of your planted foot. This will get you used to the top of movement for each side and prepare your active muscle groups for the continued movement.

This exercise is called "Speed skater" because it mimics the movement of a skater moving in a straight line but in a stationary position.

Squat jacks (Explosive)

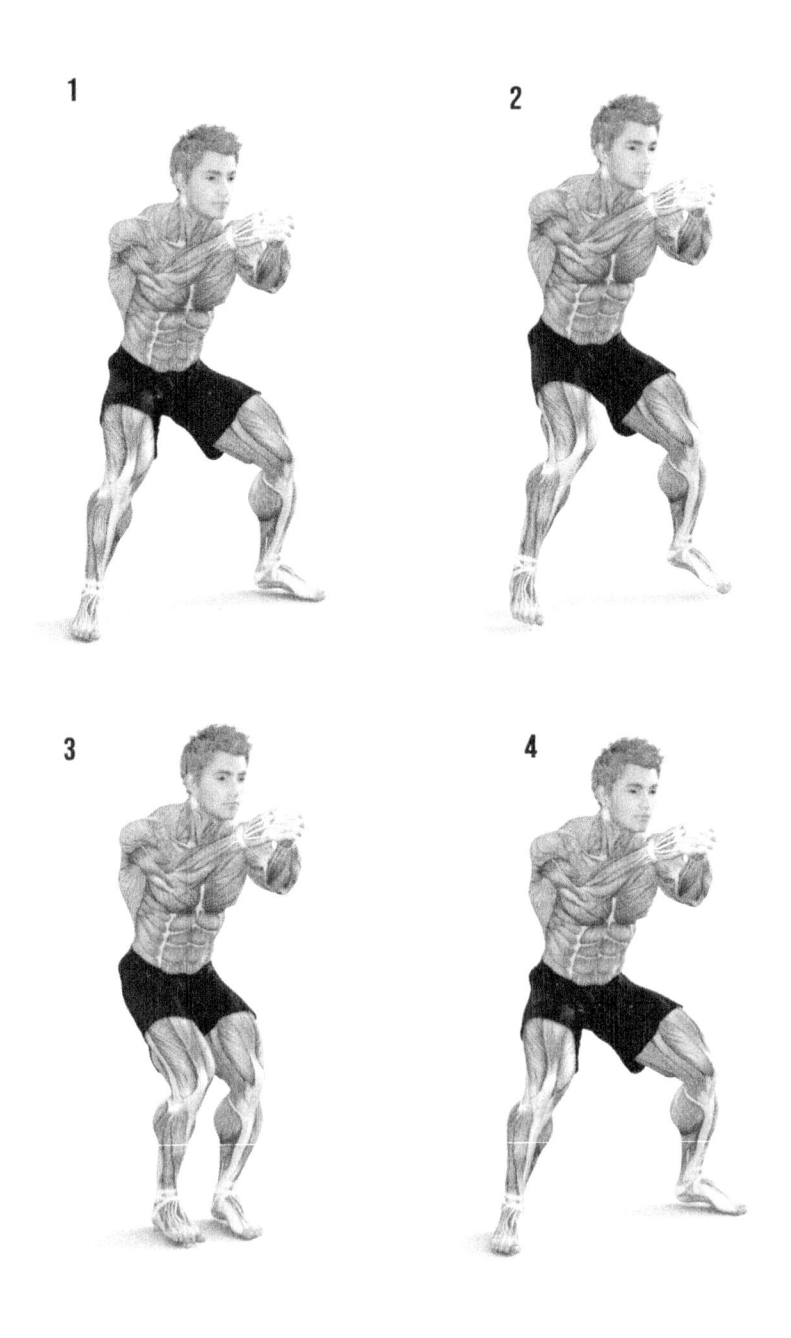

- This is an explosive movement
- Stand with your feet firmly planted on the floor at a spacing that's just past shoulder width
- Bend at the knees slightly to place you into a shallow squat position
- Bring your hands up and together to your front. This will help with balance
- As you exhale, perform a shallow jump, pushing evenly through the fronts of your feet
- As your feet leave the ground, bring them together, towards the mid line of your body
- When your feet make contact with the floor again, they should be close together
- As soon as you land, perform a shallow jump again, pushing evenly through the fronts of your feet. As your feet leave the ground, move them out towards your sides
- When your feet hit the ground, you should be in the start position again

When performing this exercise, you should maintain the shallow squat position throughout the movement and the exercise should be performed continuously. This exercise and others like it tend to work well as part of a timed set or circuit and it's a great option for a fat burning and lower body toning exercise.

This exercise can be performed at lower speeds, but we will get the most benefit in terms of fat loss and muscle tone if we perform a jump every second; one second to jump and put our feet together and one second to jump to move our feet back to the start position.

Burpees – (Explosive)

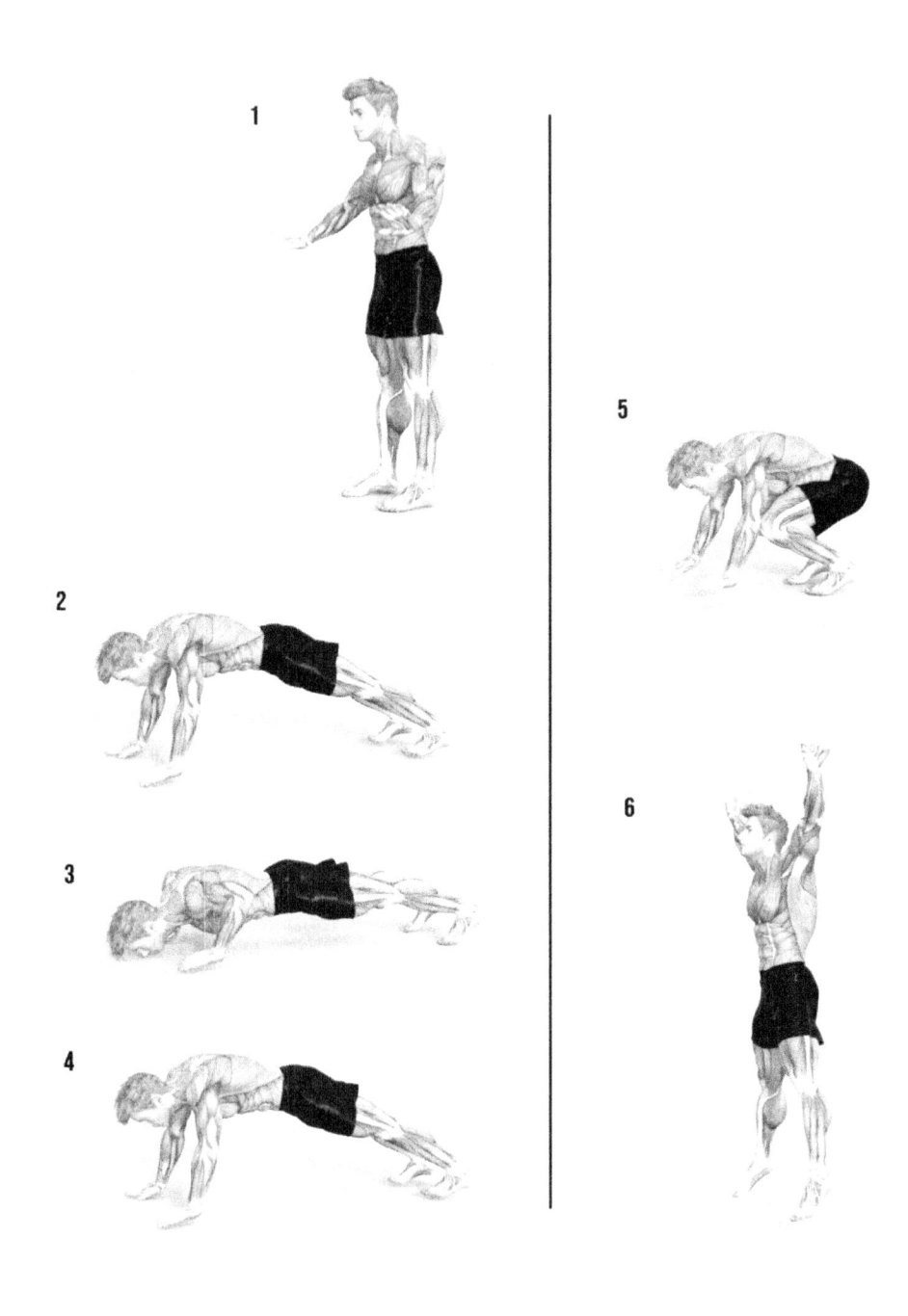

- This is an explosive movement
- From a standing position, assume the push up starting position; Palms flat on the floor about shoulder width apart and in line with your mid chest. Your back should be flat and toes planted firmly on the ground
- Perform a single push up by bending at the elbows to lower your upper body towards the floor. Keep your back flat whilst doing this
- As soon as you have returned to the push up start position, perform a squat thrust by pushing through your toes to bend your knees, bringing your knees towards your chest
- From this position, transfer your bodyweight evenly between your feet as you move to a crouching position. Your hands should not be in contact with the floor at this point
- When your full bodyweight has been transferred through the mid parts of your feet, push through the fronts of your feet as you stand up straight to perform a jump
- As you jump, ensure that you achieve a fully upright position with your back as you bring your straight arms out to your sides and above your head. Whilst doing this, simultaneously bring your feet to your sides
- Prepare for landing by bringing your feet closer together and be ready to bend your knees as you hit the floor to absorb the shock
- Immediately repeat this process until you have completed your set

Burpees is an excellent exercise for fat burning and full body muscle conditioning. In my opinion, this exercise is the top choice in this book for a "single exercise workout" as it ticks lots of boxes when it comes to aspects of fitness; muscle toning, fat burning, cardio vascular and power development.

If we break it down, a single repetition is a push up, a squat thrust and a star jump, so if you are new to this exercise and wish to add it to your routine, you should become comfortable performing these exercises first.

This is a challenging exercise for most, especially at higher repetition or time ranges. It's common to fatigue after a few repetitions, so we must be aware of our body position throughout. Watch for back arch during the push up phase, rounded back and low arms during the start jump phase. Also, when getting into the pushup position, this should be done quickly to keep the flow of the exercise, but we should take care not to throw ourselves into this position to limit impact on the shoulders.

Hand walk – (Controlled)

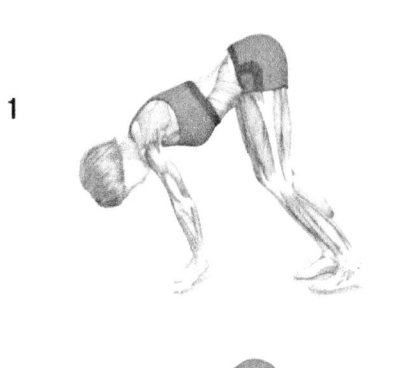

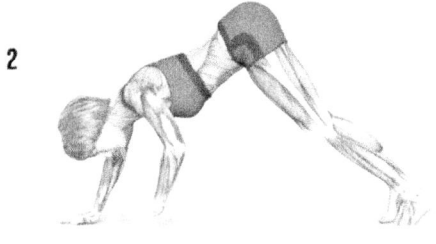

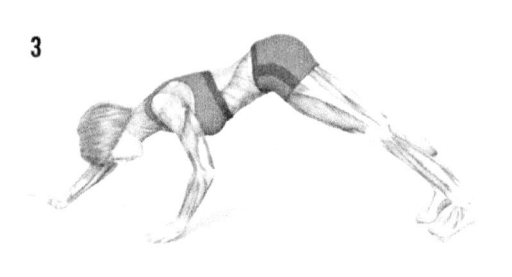

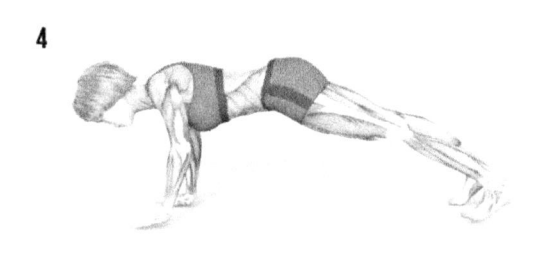

1

2

3

4

- This is a controlled movement
- Start from a standing position, hinge forward at the hips, bend at the knees slightly to place your fingertips on the floor in front of you
- You should aim to touch the floor with your fingertips as close to your toes as possible while keeping your back flat and head in a neutral position
- Once you are confident that you can transfer your upper bodyweight onto your hands, slowly tilt forward until your palms are flat on the floor
- From this position, shift your upper bodyweight to your right hand before lifting your left hand away from the floor
- Place your left hand further forward before planting it firmly on the floor
- Shift your upper bodyweight onto your left hand and mirror your previous movement with your right hand
- Continue this pattern until you reach the full push up start position. Hold for a second before reversing the process

This exercise is fairly advanced as it is lengthy and requires a good foundation of upper body strength. When "stepping forward" or reversing the "hand stepping process" it can be tempting to move one hand further than the other. This dilutes the exercise as it will require fewer steps in order to complete the exercise. It can also mean that we end up with an imbalance in strength development as we may be doing more work with one side of our body than the other.

So when performing the steps on this exercise, we should always move each hand to match the other in distance as we step. Another point to be aware of is that we should always keep our back flat and make sure we do not tilt from side to side as we step.

Quick Workouts for Busy Schedules

This section is where we get to work! There are several exercise routines set out that you can follow directly or modify to suit your individual needs, and indeed your fitness level.

There are several ways to perform a quick, effective workout, so before you get right into it, have a look at the different options.

The tonne:

I've named this exercise method "The tonne" because it is based on performing a limited amount of repetitions per exercise and does not directly take into account the time taken to complete the workout. The tonne should have ten exercise choices which should be performed in succession and without a break between exercises. Ten repetitions of each exercise should be performed. Once we have finished the last repetition of the last exercise on our list, we can rest for a short period and repeat or finish the workout.

This is an excellent choice for the beginner to exercise routines, as ten repetitions of each movement is more often than not, an achievable goal (exercise choice dependant). At the end of a single run through the exercise list, the trainer has achieved one hundred exercise repetitions altogether. This can also carry the bonus of a high sense of achievement for some trainers, which helps with motivation and mind-set.

** A point to note when following a "tonne" routine – If an exercise choice on your list has alternate movement, such as "standing side crunch", "windmill", "kickbacks" etc. You have options:

Option 1 (Recommended) - Count a single repetition for performing the exercise in both directions, or in some cases, with both sides of the body. Technically, depending on how many of these exercise choices you have in your routine, you may perform well over one hundred repetitions, but the benefits far outweigh the technicalities.

Option 2 – Count each repetition that you perform, whether it's an alternate movement or not and stick to the one hundred repetition rule to complete the workout. I would advise this option for those who are absolute beginners. It is important to train with balance, so if an exercise has an alternate pattern, it should always be performed in both directions or with both sides of the body where possible.

Timed:

Working within a timeframe is an excellent approach for beginners and advanced trainers. The most effective way to approach timed training is to create an exercise list or use one of the pre-made routines in this book and allocate a time slot to each exercise. Each exercise on the list is performed according to our chosen time slot, and all exercises on the list are performed consecutively without a rest period until the list is complete.

There are some great benefits in training this way. The first is that we can start at a shorter time allotment for each exercise and as we become stronger, fitter, and more capable of executing our workout, we can add increments of time to each exercise. This is an excellent way to track progression.

A beginner may select ten exercises to add to their workout and decide on a time frame of twenty seconds for each exercise. If they are consistent with their routine, they may be able to add an extra ten seconds to each exercise every week.

I am a big advocate of timed training, but there is a trap that people can fall into that will slow down progression and fitness results. If you do wish to try this type of training out, you should be aware of this and keep it at the forefront of your mind throughout your training sessions.

The trap that we can fall into is to slow the movements or intended cadence of the exercise down. For most trainers, there will be specific exercises in their list that are more challenging than others. It's human nature to try and make things easier, so it is very tempting while training to a time frame to run the clock down with slower movements.

Single exercise workouts:

Depending on the choice of exercise, a single movement performed every day for a set time or set number of repetitions can be very rewarding. A single exercise workout is exactly what is says on the tin. We would choose an exercise and use this for our entire workout. The best types of exercise for this are explosive, full body movements like burpees. It is possible, however, to use other more concentrated movements for single exercise workouts, but this would be more appropriate for trainers wishing to only strengthen, or improve mobility in specific areas.

Full body exercises such as burpees will engage most of our major muscle groups and as it is an explosive exercise, it will also develop our cardio vascular system.

Our single exercise workout could be performed with a set number of repetitions in mind or within an allotted timeframe. I would recommend that where possible, it is performed with a set number of repetitions from the outset.

Staying with the example of burpees as our exercise choice, our workout could be to perform one hundred repetitions every day. This would be a very short workout, but extremely intensive. We would be developing strength, power, and mobility throughout our bodies while burning a huge amount of calories and giving our cardiovascular system a demanding workout.

We wouldn't even need an exercise card for this, but it may be useful to make one in order to make notes after each session. It's useful to note where we started to struggle, and which elements of the training where most challenging during the workout. We might find that at around twenty repetitions, the push up part of the exercise became too challenging, or that we found we were totally out of breath at around ten repetitions.

We may not even finish our planned amount of repetitions due to muscle fatigue. If this happens, most may see this as a negative, or a failure, but it is actually a positive and a big win. If this happens, we have found our current limit and can set goals for progression.

If you wish to try this type of training, I have created a workout card for you to use or take inspiration from and create your own version. The card is featured later in the guide and in the "Blank exercise cards" at the back of the book.

Supersets

Supersets are two exercises performed back to back. Supersets can be used in many variations and for different fitness goals, from bodybuilding to endurance training. Traditionally, supersets were used to target opposing muscle groups during resistance training; an exercise was performed for the chest (a chest press) and immediately after an exercise was performed for the back (a row). Or an exercise was performed for the bicep (bicep curl) and immediately after, an exercise for the triceps (tricep push down).

There are several reasons that trainers might want to use supersets, and some theories about fitness benefits, but for the purpose of this guide, the main benefit is to break down a potentially unachievable workout to render it achievable, whilst also keeping the workout short and sharp.

If we decide on a list of ten challenging exercises for our workout sessions but find the sequence hard to complete, we may want to break it down by adding in rest periods throughout the program. The simplest way to do this is to perform the first two exercises on our list back to back, then have a short rest before performing the next two, and so on until we have completed all the exercises on our list.

The rest period can range from thirty seconds to two minutes, but it should be our aim to try and lower this rest period over time.

I would advise absolute beginners to consider using supersets in their workouts as it gives an unconditioned body an easier time when transitioning into a regular training routine and can also be used in conjunction with "The tonne". Intermediate trainers may also consider using supersets when upgrading their routine to include more challenging exercises. Supersets can be performed using a time frame or a repetition range.

Your Workouts Your Way

The pre-made workout routines are an excellent way to start training with this particular style. If you follow them, you will quickly begin to identify your fitness level, along with strengths and weaknesses you may have. This is a valuable step when it comes to fitness progression. But we have to remember that everyone is different. It may be that one trainer has trouble with a single exercise choice in one of the pre-made routines so switches it out for a more suitable choice, but another trainer might struggle with several movements, so more editing to the routine is needed for them.

Exercise choices are one variable we can change up in a routine, but the method is another. Following on from the last section, we will look at some other examples of exercise routines using the same exercises already mentioned, but used in a different way. Once you are familiar with the exercise choices and training methods, have a go at any of these examples. There may be a certain style that you prefer!

Superset card

SUPERSET	

ROUTINE #	

EXERCISE	REPS/ TIME
Stationary march	30 secs
Push ups on knees	
Rest	20 secs
Arm circles	30 secs
Punch it out	
Rest	20 secs
Cross over lunge	30 secs
Windmill	
Rest	20 secs
Shoulder reach	30 secs
Leg swing (front back)	

WEEKS	MON	TUE	WED	THURS	FRI	SAT	SUN
1	*	*		*	*		
2	*	*		*	*		
3	*	*		*	*		
4	*	*		*	*	*	
5	*	*		*	*	*	
6	*	*		*	*	*	

SUPERSET

ROUTINE #

EXERCISE	REPS/TIME
Tuck Jump	30 secs
Burpees	
Rest	20 secs
Tuck Jump	30 secs
Burpees	
Rest	20 secs
Tuck Jump	30 secs
Burpees	
Rest	20 secs
Tuck Jump	30 secs
Burpees	

WEEKS	MON	TUE	WED	THURS	FRI	SAT	SUN
1	*	*		*	*		
2	*	*		*	*		
3	*	*		*	*		
4	*	*		*	*	*	
5	*	*		*	*	*	
6	*	*		*	*	*	

The tonne card

THE TONNE - BEGINNER		
ROUTINE #		

EXERCISE	REPS
Stationary march	
Push ups on knees	
Arm circles	
Punch it out	
Cross over lunge	**10**
Kickbacks	
Shoulder reach	
Leg swing (front back)	
Windmill	
Standing side crunch	

WEEKS	MON	TUE	WED	THURS	FRI	SAT	SUN
1	*	*		*	*		
2	*	*		*	*		
3	*	*		*	*		
4	*	*		*	*	*	
5	*	*		*	*	*	
6	*	*		*	*	*	

Single exercise

SINGLE EXERCISE		
ROUTINE #		

EXERCISE	REPS
Burpees	
Notes: First session: Strong until 10 reps! Exhaustion at 20 reps due to cardio level. Second session: Strong until 10 reps! Exhaustion at 25 reps. Cardio level improving…	**100**

WEEKS	MON	TUE	WED	THURS	FRI	SAT	SUN
1	*	*		*	*		
2	*	*		*	*		
3	*	*		*	*		
4	*	*		*	*	*	
5	*	*		*	*	*	
6	*	*		*	*	*	

Progression modifiers

Once you have been training consistently with the same workload for a period of time, you will find that your workouts will become less challenging. This is called the "training effect". It doesn't mean that your workouts become easier; it means you have become fitter. At this point, you can carry on as you are, or you can add some progression modifiers. If you carry on as you are, your fitness progression will slow down. I like to call this "maintenance mode". There is absolutely nothing wrong with maintenance mode, in fact I think it is a great place to be once you are happy with your progress.

On the other side of this coin, if you find the workouts are getting less challenging, or dare I say "easy", and you are still not where you want to be in terms of body composition, strength, stamina, etc. Then you can consider adding some progression modifiers to your workouts. A progression modifier is something that adds extra challenge. These modifiers can be very subtle or very extreme. I would always advise that any modifiers added are towards the subtle side of this scale. In the majority of people and in my experience, it's far better to add progression modifiers that are subtle as you progress, as these changes can be made more often and your body will recover and adapt quicker. This way, the upgraded workouts will not turn into something totally different from what they have been. Think of progression modifiers at exercise tuning, rather than a new workout. Here are some options for modifiers that you might consider:

Exercise choices

- Add a new exercise to your existing workout – Adding a new exercise to your routine will give you fitness challenges that you may not have had before such as new muscle groups being used or extra workload for specific muscle groups.
- Upgrade an exercise – There are several upgrades that can be made to specific exercises mentioned in this book. Rather than add an exercise to a workout, we can choose an upgrade. For example, "Push ups on knees" can be upgraded to "Full push ups" or "Stationary march" could be upgraded to "Uppercut march". By using this modifier, your workouts will also remain in the same timeframe.

Sets repetitions

- Add more repetitions to exercises – More repetitions can be added to every exercise in the workout, or you can cherry pick which exercises you would like to increase the repetitions on. By increasing the rep range on every exercise in workout by an extra 2 – 4 reps sometimes feels insignificant, but if we are training from a routine that consists of 10 exercises and we are doing 3 sets, we would be doing an additional 60 – 120 repetitions per workout.
- Add another set to your workout – This is an upgrade that is on the more extreme side, especially if you have a lot of exercises and reps per exercise in your routine. To add this modifier, simply repeat all the exercises on your list by performing the same amount of repetitions per exercise an additional time per workout.

Time

- Increase the time you spend on exercises – If you are working from a "timed" routine, you can add several seconds to each exercise, or to specific exercises on your list. This is similar to increasing the rep range in that by increasing your time by 5 – 10 seconds per exercise will have a bigger effect on your workload than you may think.

As mentioned, I would advise adding progression modifiers in small increments, and only one at a time, especially for newer trainers. If you are training regularly and consistently, reviewing and applying them on a weekly basis is a sound plan for continued fitness progression. The obvious catch for adding more exercises, sets, reps and time spent on each exercise is the increased overall time spent working out. But the more time we spend with an elevated heart rate, the more calories we burn, and so the better the fitness benefits. Due to the nature of the training styles and exercise choices highlighted in this guide, however, a twenty to thirty minute workout can be very intense. This timeframe is still considered a quick workout.

Some free stuff?

If you would like to learn more about this series and my other books, you can do so by visiting my author page. Visit Amazon and search "James Atkinson".

You can stay up to date with my current activities, be alerted to deeply discounted, or free new release by signing up to my email list. When you sign up, there are a couple of short PDF guides related to diet and exercise that you may find useful. These get delivered as part of the sign-up process.

As we all know, diet plays a big part in health and fitness, and the two subjects fit hand in hand. So I would like to offer you a free download of seven healthy recipes that I created and use regularly myself. You can copy the recipes exactly, add your own twist to them, or simply take inspiration from them.

If you would like to grab this along with other free content such as video tutorials, motivation and fitness planning guides become a part of my email list and we'll reach our fitness goals together! You can do so by following the link below, or using the QR code.

https://yourfitnesssuccess.com/all-the-freebiees/

Don't worry, I never spam, and newsletters are infrequent, but there is always something of value inside when they are sent.

Conclusion and Next Steps

Quick workouts performed as this guide highlights will give everyone the chance for fitness progression, including fat loss, muscle tone, cardio vascular health and increases in strength and stamina provided that consistency with regular, challenging training is undertaken.

I hope this guide has been useful and, as always, I'm more than happy to answer any questions that you may have. If something is not as clear as you would like, you have questions about planning your routine etc. Please feel free to ask for help. Give me a shout at **admin@yourfitnesssuccess.com** and I'll do my best to help where I can.

There is much that can be done in terms of fitness progression in or out of a gym environment. With a bit of knowledge and a few tools, we can work towards any fitness goal and reach our potential with health and fitness. We can even merge bodyweight training with resistance band training or add in a few barbell and dumbbell exercises to really tailor our plans to precisely fit our personal goals.

Other guides I have published that are written in a similar format to this one may help you with inspiration and take your training to the next level. If you found this and any of the other guides useful, it would help me out more than you know if you returned to the store you bought it from and left a short review on the sales page. I'd be eternally grateful for this! You can even review this particular title by clicking or scanning the QR code below.

You can find my other guides by searching "James Atkinson" at your online bookstore.

Thanks for your interest and I wish you all the best!

Jim

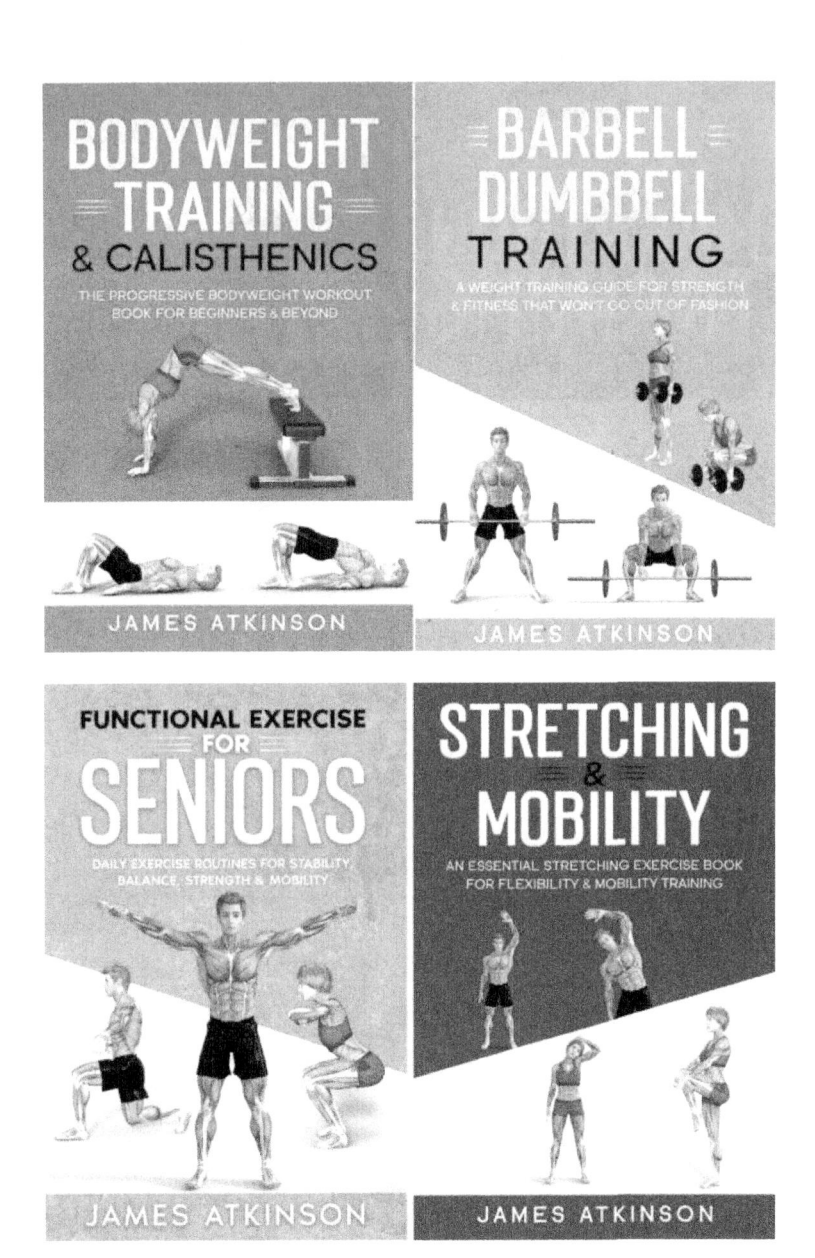

Standard

ROUTINE #	

EXERCISE	SETS	REPS / TIME

WEEKS	MON	TUE	WED	THURS	FRI	SAT	SUN
1							
2							
3							
4							
5							
6							

ROUTINE #	

EXERCISE	SETS	REPS / TIME

WEEKS	MON	TUE	WED	THURS	FRI	SAT	SUN
1							
2							
3							
4							
5							
6							

Single exercise

SINGLE EXERCISE		
ROUTINE #		

EXERCISE	REPS
Notes:	

WEEKS	MON	TUE	WED	THURS	FRI	SAT	SUN
1							
2							
3							
4							
5							
6							

SINGLE EXERCISE

ROUTINE #	

EXERCISE	REPS
Notes:	

WEEKS	MON	TUE	WED	THURS	FRI	SAT	SUN
1							
2							
3							
4							
5							
6							

The Tonne

THE TONNE - BEGINNER	

ROUTINE #		

EXERCISE	REPS
	10

WEEKS	MON	TUE	WED	THURS	FRI	SAT	SUN
1							

THE TONNE - BEGINNER

ROUTINE #

EXERCISE	REPS
	10

WEEKS	MON	TUE	WED	THURS	FRI	SAT	SUN
1							
2							
3							
4							
5							
6							

Video course

If you found this guide helpful and you are a beginner to weight loss and exercise, I have something that might help you!

My genuine passion as a fitness professional is helping the beginner earn their first actual results. This stage of the journey can be truly life changing. I have always empathised with the feeling of not being able to get where we want to be. I also know the feeling of overwhelm when there's too much information on a subject. So I created a video course that any beginner can follow from their own home. Just press the play button and we both train together!

We will work on a weekly basis, the first week is really an important week where we lay the foundations, we'll sit down and start planning for success, well find our motivation, get specific about our goals, I always advise making these goals ambitious because we can all achieve more than we think we can!

Week 1 through to week 6 is where we hit our home workouts! Each week is more progressive than the last. We build on our training from the previous week by tweaking the exercise choices, adding intensity and further challenging ourselves. Some people develop quicker and can move from week to week seamlessly, but the beauty of this course is that if you find a week a bit too challenging, you can repeat the previous week. Everyone moves at a different pace so it's no problem!

So if this sounds like something you are interested in, please check out the video testimonials, check out the sample videos and you can even start the course for free!

It would be great to see you over at:

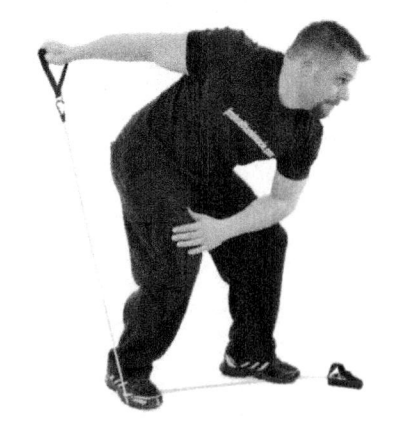

YourFitnessSuccess.com

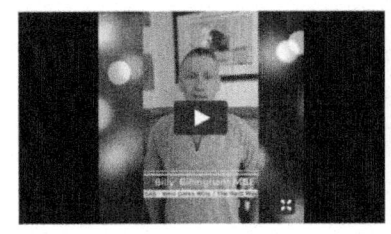

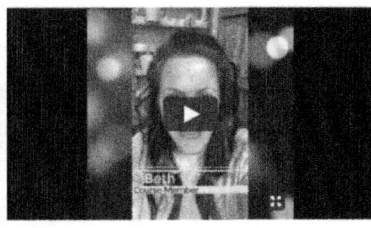

"Far more than your usual fitness video training! This is a serious, progressive exercise course!"

YOURFITNESSSUCCESS.COM

PAPERBACK EDITION

PUBLISHED BY: JBA Publishing

http://www.yourfitnesssuccess.com

admin@yourfitnesssuccess.com

Quick workouts real results

Copyright © 2024 by James Atkinson

All Rights Reserved.

No part of this book may be reproduced or transmitted in any form or by any means, electronic, mechanical, photocopying, recording, or otherwise, without the prior written permission of James Atkinson, except for brief quotations in critical reviews or articles.

Requests for permission to make copies of any part of this book should be submitted to James Atkinson at admin@yourfitnesssuccess.com

DISCLAIMER

Although the author and publisher have made every effort to ensure that the information contained in this book was accurate at the time of release, the author and publisher do not assume and hereby disclaim any liability to any party for any loss, damage, or disruption caused by errors or omissions in this book, whether such errors or omissions result from negligence, accident, or any other cause.

First published in 2024

Printed in Great Britain
by Amazon